HIGH PERFORMANCE HAIR

McGRAW-HILL BOOK COMPANY
New York St. Louis San Francisco Hamburg Mexico Toronto

HIGH

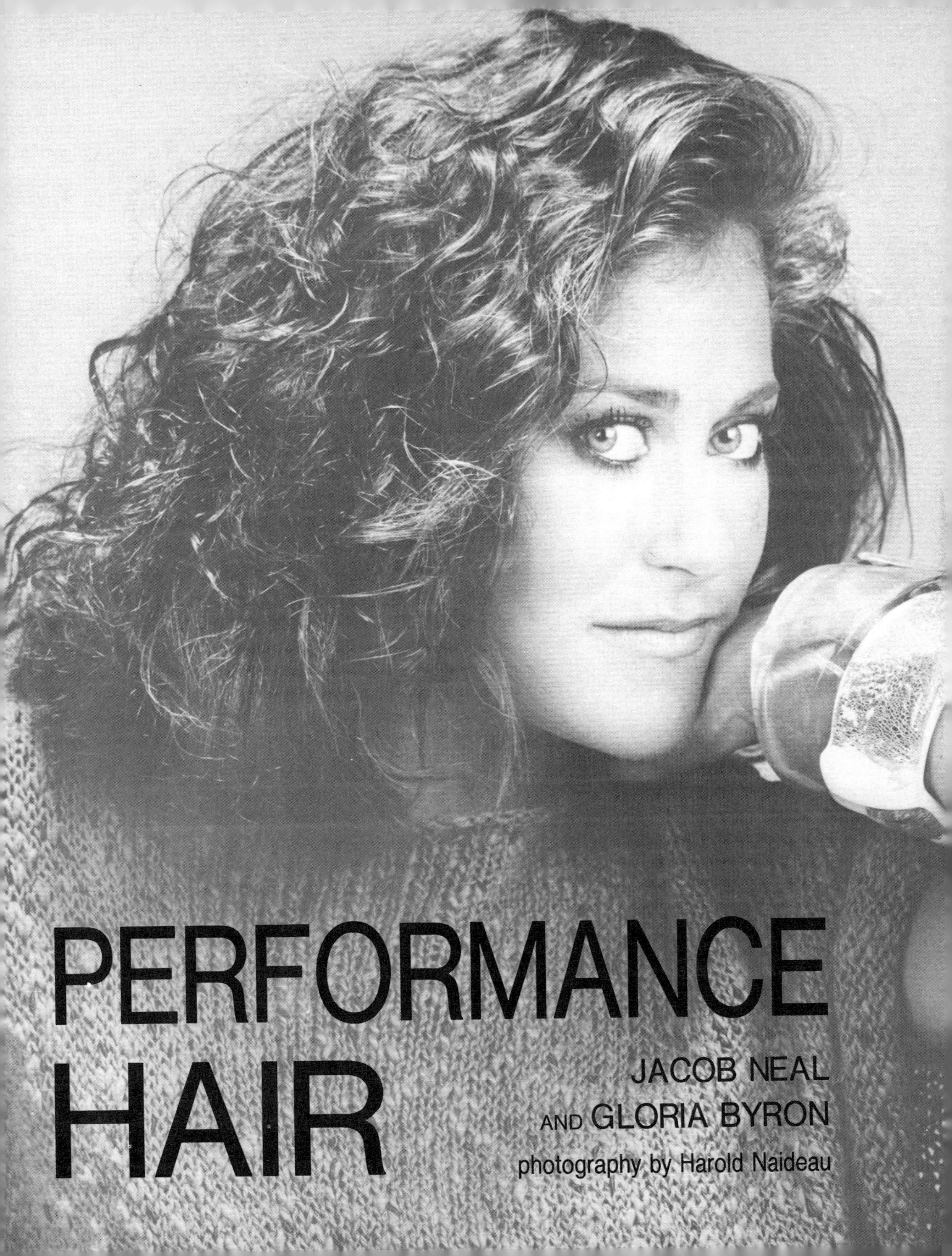

PERFORMANCE HAIR

JACOB NEAL AND GLORIA BYRON

photography by Harold Naideau

ILLUSTRATIONS BY MARY DICHITO

CREDITS:

Suzy Chaffee: Lydia Milars, Make-up.

Nancy Lieberman: Lydia Milars, Make-up.

April Allen: Lydia Milars, Make-up; Jim Woodmansey, Fashion Stylist.

Leslie Allen: Lydia Milars, Make-up; Jim Woodmansey, Fashion Stylist.

Martina Navratilova: Tom Murphy, Make-up; Jim Woodmansey, Fashion Stylist.

Jennifer Chandler: Christopher Cook, Make-up; Amy Glenn, Fashion Stylist.

Candy Costie: Christopher Cook, Make-up; Amy Glenn, Fashion Stylist.

Debi Thomas: Christopher Cook, Make-up; Amy Glenn, Fashion Stylist.

Hollis Stacy: Tom Murphy, Make-up; Jim Woodmansey, Fashion Stylist.

Gladys Portugues: Tom Murphy, Make-up; Lisa Emett, Fashion Stylist.

Judy Blumberg: Tom Murphy, Make-up; Lisa Emett, Fashion Stylist.

Muffin Spencer-Devlin: Susan Amer, Make-up; Jim Woodmansey, Fashion Stylist.

Denise Austin: Tom Murphy, Make-up; Jim Woodmansey, Fashion Stylist.

Chris Evert Lloyd: Susan Amer, Make-up; Jim Woodmansey, Fashion Stylist.

Gloria Byron and Jacob Neal: Susan Amer, Make-up.

BOOK DESIGN BY PATRICE FODERO

9 8 7 6 5 4 3 2

For my parents, Sonia and Paul, whose love and pride gave me the determination to become the best I can be.

J. N.

ACKNOWLEDGMENTS

We wish to thank:

* our agent, Ivy Fischer Stone of Fifi Oscard Associates, who recognized instantly that our book was rich with possibilities, and our editors, P. J. Haduch and Tom Miller, who helped us turn the idea into reality.

*Rhonda Racz, who orchestrated our collaboration, Phyllis Klein, Jim Essey and Lorraine Ewing of Clairol, who generously shared their expertise, Joseph Virgilio and Lynn Barrett, Holly Turner of the Women's Sports Foundation, Paula Marafino of the Ladies Professional Golf Association, Peggy Gossett of the Women's Tennis Association, and Mary Healy of Milady Publishing Company.

We especially want to express our deep appreciation to the athletes featured in HIGH PERFORMANCE HAIR. Without their participation this book would not have been possible.

I would like to extend a special thanks to Michael-Jon Boone, who taught me his brilliant techniques of hairdressing, Valerie Viglione, whose head of hair remains a constant challenge and inspiration to my career, Louise Cotter, who has always made her wealth of knowledge in the hairdressing industry available to me, Allan Kalmus and Alexis McCormick, who believed there was more to me than a pair of scissors, Elizabeth McCarthy for figuring out how much more there was, and what to do with it, and Allyn Seidman from Clairol for harnessing all my energy and giving it direction.

Jacob Neal

I offer special thanks to my husband Stuart and my daughters Linda and Lisa for their loving support and encouragement.

Gloria Byron

CONTENTS

FOREWORD

In September 1982, while traveling the Ladies Professional Golf Association (LPGA) Tour as hairstylist to many of the top women golfers, Jacob Neal took time out to contribute his considerable talent to the women athletes gathered at the Plaza Hotel in New York for the Women's Sports Foundation's annual awards program, "A Salute to Women in Sports." Since then he has remained a permanent and popular fixture at that event and at the foundation's West Coast awards program.

The women athletes line up and wait for hours during the afternoon prior to the black-tie dinner in order to have Jacob cut, style, reshape, or update their hair and to get his advice on maintaining those hairstyles on their own. Many athletes have become his faithful clients, calling on him every time their travel brings them to New York.

Perhaps the most significant difference between Jacob and other hairdressers who have cared for these women's hair is his ability to teach them how to do what he does, showing them how to use mousses, gels, and other styling tools so they can easily re-create the looks he has given them and innovate a few of their own.

As internationally known sportswomen they experience constant exposure to stresses that are a lot tougher on their appearances than those confronting most other workingwomen. If they can develop a facility for managing their own hair successfully, despite their almost nonstop schedules and the other occupational hazards inherent in sports, you can, too. In *High Performance Hair,* with coauthor Gloria Byron, Jacob Neal shows you how. Written in a lively entertaining style, the book is fun to read and easy to follow. And whether you indulge in sports or knock yourself out simply keeping up with the demands of career, social life, and family life, you'll appreciate the trade secrets Jacob shares, enabling you to take full charge of your own looks. For with his helpful advice, you'll learn how to acquire and maintain beautiful, healthy hair that makes you look and feel like a winner in every sense of the word.

Holly Turner
Associate Director
Women's Sports Foundation

ONE

GETTING OFF ON THE RIGHT TRACK: YOUR OWN SIGNATURE

Have you ever wished you could look like Linda Evans, Christie Brinkley, Jaclyn Smith, or some other famous beauty? Why fantasize when your own reflection can make you feel that every other woman should want to look like you?

Another dream? Perhaps—but with a big difference: This one stands a far better chance of coming true—particularly if yours is a hectic life-style filled with intellectual pastimes and managing a career, a household and a family, perhaps with sports and other regular exercise thrown in.

Even if only part of the whirlwind I described here resembles your way of life, this book was written for you. In it I'll show you the relatively simple moves I think you need to master to turn that dream into reality. But equally important, I'll explain how to eliminate all the unnecessary and expensive primping frills that seem to eat up your time, discouraging you from bothering to try.

Obviously most budgets and busy schedules also preclude time and funds for the professional pampering that's all in a day's work (and is tax-deductible besides) for models and women in show business. After all, they have a gaggle of wardrobe mistresses, makeup artists, and hairstylists standing by to help them put their best selves forward—at least for however long it takes the lens to capture the "flawless" images you admire.

Ideally you, too, could use a boost from that kind of "natural beauty." With fitness high in the public consciousness these days, and physical exercise of every sort woven into the fabric of our lives, you, like so many modern women, may well move to the swing of a golf club, to the staccato of ball against racket, the swoosh of skis on slopes, the beat of aerobic dance music, or your own rhythmic breathing as you bend and stretch in pursuit of a healthy body. Even if you prefer a somewhat more sedentary existence, more than likely you burn up a fair amount of energy just trying to stay on top of all you have to do—at work, at home, for others, and for that special person who always seems to get short shrift: yourself. Just imagine the havoc this kind of perpetual-motion life-style can play with your appearance and grooming routine.

But you don't have to imagine, do you? If you're active, you already experience the all too frequent showering and shampooing that tend to dry out your hair and skin. Then you repeatedly hit your hair with heat from a dryer and maybe from electric rollers as well. And these assaults often come only after your hair and skin have already endured the effects of sun, wind, rain, heat, cold, or whatever punishment nature sees fit to inflict when you venture outdoors.

Then there's the nuisance of applying and reapplying makeup during the course of a day—that is, if you have time when rushing from workout to work or wherever. Most active women I know say they feel lucky just to look tidy and tranquil much of the time, let alone like their "ideal" concepts of beauty.

Granted, many Hollywood and Madison Avenue stars have been more than willing to share their beauty and fitness secrets. Perhaps your favorite is among them. But how can you hope to duplicate her results without her hair, skin tone, and bone structure? Actually, even if you resembled her, how could you maintain the perfection you perceive in her appearance without the frequent attention of the beauty, fashion, and fitness experts she very likely retains? You probably couldn't.

But you can turn your own natural resources into a look you love—one that makes you feel admired, even envied. And you can maintain it quickly and efficiently with only occasional help from personal-care pros. However, to sustain yourself through some of the most difficult days and trying situations, you must, above all, *gain control over your hair,* which draws immediate attention to you. This is the component of the beauty ritual that seems to frustrate women more than most other aspects of grooming. Count how many times you've said in sheer exasperation, "Ugh, this hair! I can't do a thing with it."

That's where I come in. As hairstylist and beauty consultant to some of the world's foremost female athletes—who experience far more physical stress than most other workingwomen, including those who labor strictly in the home—I'll teach you a variety of high performance/low maintenance beauty techniques I use in their behalf and have *taught them to use.* They include simple approaches to hair care and styling that will forever banish the belief that your active way of life must complicate your grooming routine or restrict you to a few boring drip-dry haircuts.

The only issue will be how far you must depart from your natural state to get the look you want. The more you have to do to make your hair or your other features bend to your will, the more time-consuming and discouraging your efforts. And since my purpose is to encourage you, I won't be giving you any low maintenance tips for such radical changes as turning dark brown hair pale blond. They don't exist. Instead, you'll get the kind of hair help and beauty advice I give to golf luminaries like Nancy Lopez and Hollis Stacy, tennis star Martina Navratilova, and Suzy Chaffee, an Olympic and world champion free style skier turned actress and businesswoman, just to name a few of my better-known clients who indulge in at least as many strenuous activities as you do. In my book that means expending the smallest amount of time and effort to do the most you can (which you'll see is quite a lot) with what you have.

I know about your superbusy days and nights, crammed to overflowing with no fewer than a million things to do, leaving you with little time, let alone energy or ambition, to fuss with your looks in any major way. Still, I'm convinced you can learn how to achieve the kind of high performance/ultra low maintenance results I'm challenging you to strive for. Once you do, you won't need lots of time to look great all the time. And with this book I hope to help you discover the enormous satisfaction to be had in meeting that challenge head-on.

First, let's explore why looking fabulous ranks high on the list of items essential to your well-being. It's simple, really! The way you look is *crucial* to making you a winner or a loser in life. Your appearance greatly influences the way you're perceived by those who can push you ahead or hold you back. It also profoundly affects the way you feel about yourself—perhaps the single most important factor, psychologists will tell you, in motivating you to strive for success or settle for mediocrity or failure.

So forget what you were taught about not judging books by their covers, beauty's penetrating only skin-deep, and other platitudes meant to make cosmetic concerns seem frivolous. I can attest to the significance of looking and feeling attractive—or unattractive—in deciding how well or poorly we do in life because I witness it in action almost every day.

Ask the women on the Ladies Professional Golf Association tour, for example, to list factors that determine their successes and failures on the circuit. Right up there along with swing and putting technique, most will mention how they look.

"If I feel I look good, I play well," Jan Stephenson, a top earner in professional golf, told a *PM Magazine* interviewer. She added that on the rare occasions when she can't pay the usual attention to her appearance, "I'm depressed all day and play badly as a result."

Stephenson, a glamorous role model to many of her fans, noted that because people watch them and some women may want to emulate them, leaders in women's sports must maintain their outward images.

Three-time U.S. Open winner, Hollis Stacy heartily agrees. Stacy points out how she won the Inamori Golf Classic in San Jose several years ago even though (or perhaps because) just before that event she focused more on how her hair looked than on the fine points of her game and says it's as important for professional golfers to look their best as it is for cover girls, particularly when their tournaments are televised.

"Somehow, when you look your best, you feel your best, so you *do* your best," she asserts, "probably because you know everyone is watching. And nothing lifts your spirits higher or gives you more confidence than knowing others appreciate how great you look."

Basketball star Nancy Lieberman, who plays swing position for the Dallas Diamonds, finds that her looks affect her concentration and attitude in competition. Lieberman, known to her fans as Lady Magic, says, "When I feel especially good about myself because I look good, I walk out on that court feeling and probably projecting a lot of self-assurance. Not only does that improve my game, but I think it intimidates my opponents a little, also working in my favor."

In one way or another these athletes are describing the extra edge of confidence you get from knowing how wonderful you look. But if you want more concrete proof that appearance can make the difference between winning and losing in life, you might consult one of the numerous physical-attractiveness studies conducted over the past decade at learning centers like Boston University and the University of Minnesota. These confirm what psychologists have asserted for years: Looking terrific on the outside makes you feel terrific on the inside. Those positive feelings tend to inspire self-confidence, vitality, and peak performance.

Much of the research shows that others tend to judge your inner characteristics, such as intelligence, capability, and sincerity, largely on how attractive you are. A 1985 television documentary demonstrated over and over again how attractive individuals often are credited with more positive traits than those considered unattractive. Good-looking people, many social scientists maintain, tend to get breaks in life frequently denied those who fall short in looks. They're more likely to be hired, they earn more money, and they move up the ladder at a faster clip.

Such reasons to look as attractive as you can hardly seem frivolous to me. Rather, they tend to explode the myth that beauty is only skin-deep.

Admittedly what "good-looking" means to you may not quite mesh with my interpretation or someone else's. But within commonly accepted standards of physical attractiveness and unattractiveness, the very fact that people differ on precisely where one ends and the other begins suggests that you have lots of room to come up a winner with what nature has given you.

The best way I know to make the most of your assets (and perhaps your liabilities, too) is to cultivate an overall look that bears your "signature," one that makes a distinctive statement about you because it reflects your values, philosophies, interests, and tastes—in short, who you are.

Start by examining the various facets of your personality and life-style. With thoughtful planning they can contribute to a statement that becomes uniquely yours. What kind of work do you do? The characteristics and aptitudes that steered you to one occupation rather than another—or the occupation itself—can provide input for (or even govern) the visual image you want to present to the world.

Catherine, a superbright fledgling banker, whose business future is high on her list of priorities, comes in to get her medium-length bobbed hair trimmed every six weeks. She's firmly convinced that to be taken seriously in the male-dominated world of high finance, she has to *appear* not only competent but successful. So she scrupulously maintains her simple but high-quality visual statement with the right hair and makeup and a relatively small but well-thought-out wardrobe.

A lot of Catherine's social life is tied to business, so even her after-five clothes don't boast much flash or dash. Instead, she favors the cool sophistication to be found in a few variations of the classic black dress—a look she often accentuates with sleek hairdos swept up or back.

On the other hand, the rebel within you could find expression in your appearance, revealing your fantasy self-image (the way you'd *like* to be perceived) or simply another side of your personality. I once knew a high school cheerleading coach who, by day, looked every inch the gym teacher she was, from her well-worn sneakers and white anklets to the length of shiny hair pulled off her face and twisted up the back of her head. But by night this female superjock, as some of her fellow teachers saw her, seemed a lot less the Olympian than a Greek goddess with that gorgeous blond hair cascading loosely about her shoulders. And she always heightened her sex appeal with the soft, fluid lines of body-tracing clothes—quite a departure from the sweat suits she often donned for work.

Of course, a distinctive and dramatic style statement could stem simply from what makes you most comfortable. The wife of a college president I know—who feels at ease only in the casual clothes that suit her life-style at the small, rustic campus—translates her favorite skirt-and-sweater look into outfits for the obligatory, sometimes formal college fundraisers she and her husband host. Long before bejeweled and beribboned sweaters and sweatshirts made fashion news for evening, she was putting together her own versions, using cashmere sweaters adorned with just the right amount of glitter and other dressy touches, such as an occasional satin or chiffon scarf to match a skirt. Her only concession to a formal hairstyle is the occasional addition of jeweled barrettes or combs in place of the plainer variety she wears for daytime.

Actually any attitude or personal preference can make the basis for a look that bears your very own signature. Do you devour Barbara Cartland novels and melt when someone sends you lacy valentines? Maybe the incurable romantic in you dreams of dancing until dawn, draped in yards of swirling chiffon, with hair falling in soft waves.

Or short, sleek, sculptured hairstyles might be more to your liking if you like crisply tailored silhouettes more than ruffles and stark white walls adorned with Art Deco better than warm wood paneling.

If camping and trout fishing constitute your idea of a great vacation, you may feel happier with patched and faded Levi's, well-worn leather jackets, and tousled hair than with the casual chic of those who go to Club Med.

Better yet, why not look tousled for your company's picnic, sleek and efficient at your next new-business presentation, and thoroughly romance-inspiring for dinner and dancing under the stars? Your on-the-go life-style shouldn't frustrate your sense of drama or your need to seem unpredictable at times any more than it should hamper your ability to create a fabulous basic look. Virtually any kind of hair can give you flexibility—depending on how cleverly you use what nature gave you.

In this book I'll show you how to gain the kind of control you'll need to vary your hair quickly and easily for different occasions. The same kind of control holds true for makeup—from your subtle daytime face to more intensely dramatic effects for dressier evening events, often attainable with little more than a flick of your wrist.

Where do you get the ideas to help you put your basic look together? From the women who epitomize active living. Even if your life-style leaves you little time or inclination to indulge in sports, *celebrated sportswomen make practical role models* for a variety of reasons:

More visible than ever before, today's sports stars have to look their best all the time, just as models and actresses do. But the reality of the full-time athlete's life-style resembles yours much more than the fantasies spun by screen stars and models.

Sports personalities pursue as livelihoods what you may well take up for occasional recreation or just to stay fit. And an athlete's looks, like yours, must withstand more rigorous tests under real-life conditions than the seemingly flawless beauty of a Victoria Principal or Joan Collins who always manages to look sensational on camera.

Let's face it, for athletes and for you "sensational" isn't enough—especially on camera—unless it can stand up to strenuous physical activity, drenching perspiration, and the ravages of sun, wind, humidity, and rain or snow. After all, you can't stop the action for cosmetic touch-ups during a tense moment at the Dinah Shore Invitational or in the middle of a frenzied rally at Wimbledon as you can on a *Dynasty* or *Dallas* set.

Touring sports stars, with their frenetic schedules, have few opportunities to seek expert grooming help, and they can afford no more time than you can for elaborate do-it-yourself techniques.

Still, even an athlete won't make a suitable star-gazing subject if you merely attempt to mimic her look. With the help of a wide range of sports celebrities featured in the book, I'll show you how to borrow problem-solving ideas from various sources and adapt them to your own special brand of beauty. The ideas can work for you whether you enjoy the sporting life or you simply want to look terrific no matter how wild your day turns out.

At one time you might have been hard-pressed to find outstanding looks to borrow from. Some of the earlier sports figures like ice skater Sonja Henie and ballet swimmer Esther Williams projected lots of glamour. But by the late forties Hollywood's version of sports beauty had been eclipsed by other concerns among female athletes. Golf notables like Babe Zaharias and Kathy Whitworth (who snagged her first of nearly ninety victories in 1959 and is still a strong player) showed more interest in ways to enhance their images as professional athletes than in trappings to boost their glamour. By the sixties the sportswoman's quest for appropriate recognition had become a crusade. Superstars like JoAnne Carner in golf and Billie Jean King in tennis, bent on stressing their ability as athletes, had put glamour on the back burner.

Those missionaries of the sixties and seventies have brought women's sports a long way. In doing so, they also paved a path for today's new breed of female athletes, who now feel freer to aim for winning combinations of ability and appearance. The result: a whole range of striking, actionworthy looks that can work as well for you as for them.

In this book I'll show you how to create some of those looks by maximizing the potential of your hair and other features and working around their limitations. I'll also cover how to select local experts you can turn to for help and how to communicate with them effectively for the results you want. I'll teach you, as I teach all my clients—famous, infamous, or anonymous—how to take charge of your appearance and master simple techniques for maintaining your high performance look within the context of your life-style. All *you* have to do is give it your personal best.

TWO

YOUR GAME PLAN

LET'S TAKE IT FROM THE TOP

This is your year to discover the joy of loving the way you look and maintaining the looks you love. You can achieve a look that will make you feel great inside, take almost no trouble, demand little time, and fit beautifully and comfortably into your active, perhaps athletic life.

No single feature can help your efforts or diminish your results more than your hair. It's the first thing people notice. From the back, your hair is *all* they see above your shoulders. Turn your head, and it becomes the frame that sets off your face. Your hair can make you seem sexy, slovenly, fascinating, or dull. It reflects the state of your health and how you feel about yourself. And since scrutinizing eyes tend to travel from the top downward, your hair, together with the face it frames, sets the tone for your total appearance.

So any statement you want to make with your physical presence clearly must begin with a lovely head of hair, cut and coiffed to suit the image you want to project and to flatter your face and figure. Your look will last only as long as your crowning glory continues to convey that image.

Judging by the popularity of role models from Rapunzel and Goldilocks to Farrah Fawcett, I'd say that from earliest childhood women recognize the impact their hair makes. Until well after the turn of the century very long hair prevailed, placing definite limits on styling options. And if you didn't look your best with all that length piled atop your head in some fashion, you were out of luck.

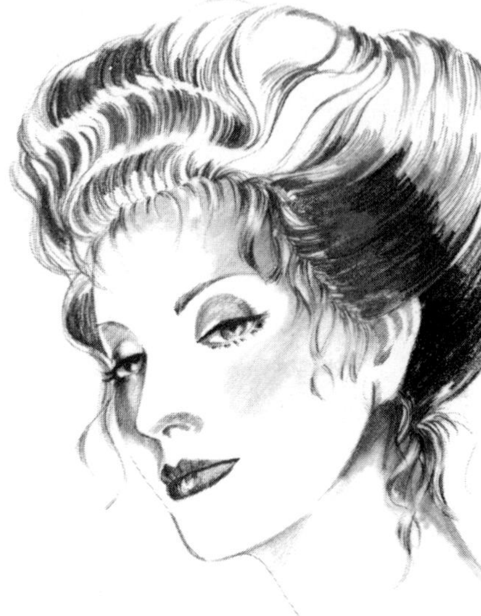

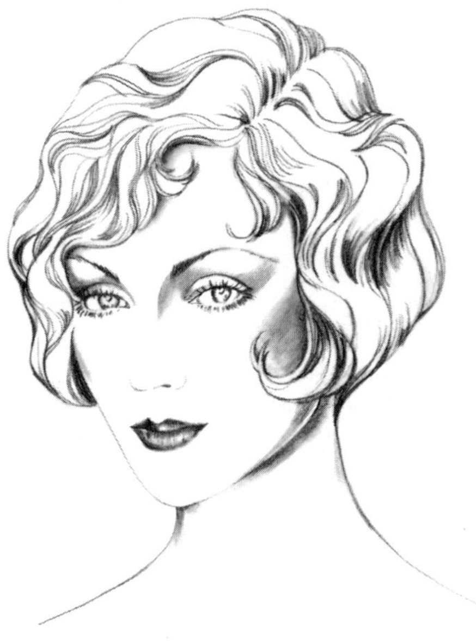

But then flappers and their bobbed hair freed women to choose from among many hair lengths to flatter their looks and to serve their changing roles. Soon more versatile and manageable hair lengths became a vehicle for self-expression women have been using ever since.

Nowhere was this more apparent than on the silver screen, where stars like Veronica Lake, whose silky blond hair dipped seductively over one eye, and Rita Hayworth, whose glorious, shiny waves cascaded about her shoulders, used hair to hype their glamour.

Even today celebrities like Tina Turner

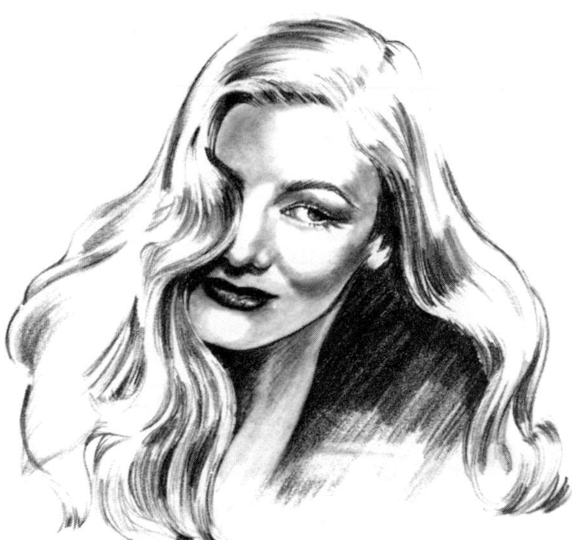

and Chaka Khan rely on hairstyles to boost their visual impact. And how many women have influenced hairstyles more than ice-skating star Dorothy Hamill? Her widely imitated wedge cut gained as much attention as her skating talents when she landed the 1976 Olympic gold medal.

Your hair can contribute to the way people see you as theirs does to our perceptions of them. But in order to achieve such results with relative ease, you must first understand what really happens when your hair behaves as it does under certain stresses.

It's a lot like maximizing your position in competitive situations no matter when they arise by assessing your opponent's strengths and weaknesses beforehand. The opponents in this case: your hair's steadfast refusal to do what you want it to without a lot of coaxing combined with a variety of stresses that encourage such stubborn behavior. The simplest way to gain this kind of foresight is by examining a single hair and evaluating the challenges it faces. Only then can you devise successful defensive strategies.

ASSESS YOUR NATURAL RESOURCES

Each hair grows out of a follicle, a tiny depression in your scalp containing several glands that secrete oil, nature's protective coating to that hair shaft. This lubricant, along with nutrients in your system, helps keep your hair elastic so it can stretch and bounce back without breaking.

Depending on your genes, the hair shaft can be curly, wavy, or straight and coarse, medium, or fine. "Fine," by the way, doesn't refer to how much hair you have. "Fine hair" simply describes a hair shaft smaller in diameter (more slender) than coarser hair. You can have abundant fine hair or sparse hair on the coarser side. Whatever its diameter, the hair shaft determines your hair's *texture,* not its thickness.

A shaft of hair has two layers (although many people have a third layer, a medulla, which serves no real purpose). The inner layer, called the *cortex,* forms the hair shaft's bulk, strength, elasticity, and color (the pigment is inside, too). The *cuticle* layer, on the surface, protects the cortex. Its appearance is often compared with fish scales or a shingled roof: overlapping scalelike cells capable of opening and closing. When those cuticles lie flat, the outer layer imparts shine to the hair.

A SUREFIRE WINNER

A superhealthy hair shaft has a richly nourished cortex, plump with just the right amount of moisture, making the hair resilient but not limp. Its smooth cuticle layer basically lies flat but lifts just a touch to add some of that fullness we call body and to let in a bit more moisture from the air. But alas, I've yet to see one. Few, if any, individuals—especially if they are active—can hope to come by such perfection naturally, if at all. In fact, nature often shares the blame for your considerably less than perfect hair.

TOO MUCH OF A GOOD THING

If, in the natural course of heredity, you wound up with baby-fine hair, you know only too well what I mean. Fine hair tends to accumulate oil fast and droops at the slightest provocation. That happens because the oil each gland secretes has a much smaller area to lubricate on the slender hair shaft. With such terrific lubrication comes one of many classic good news/bad news dilemmas common to hair: The hair shaft, less vulnerable though it may be to drying (thanks to that extra protection), simply wilts under the weight of the excess oil. You need a strategy that will reduce the oil and control it.

HAIR LEFT HIGH AND DRY

Starting at the opposite end of the spectrum also puts you at a disadvantage. Excessive dryness—which comes in part from overexposure to nature's elements—at the least creates dull, hard-to-control, flyaway hair. At worst it can produce splitting or other damage, evoking images of straw or fraying rope, as one of my clients described her problem.

Her impressions weren't far off base. The drier the hair shaft, the more brittle the cuticle layer, hampering its ability to lie flat. So, instead of looking smooth and healthy, the hair shaft tends to appear rough around the edges. And the cuticles can't adequately protect the cortex, subjecting it to even more external stresses and moisture loss. In extreme cases some of the cuticles can chip off, permanently

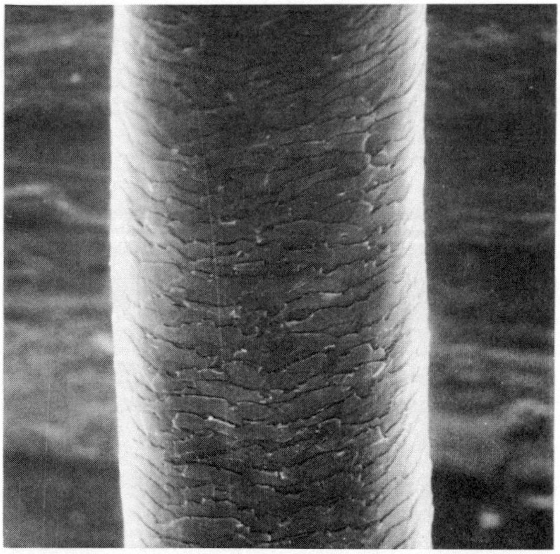

HEALTHY HAIRSHAFT (magnified 700 times)

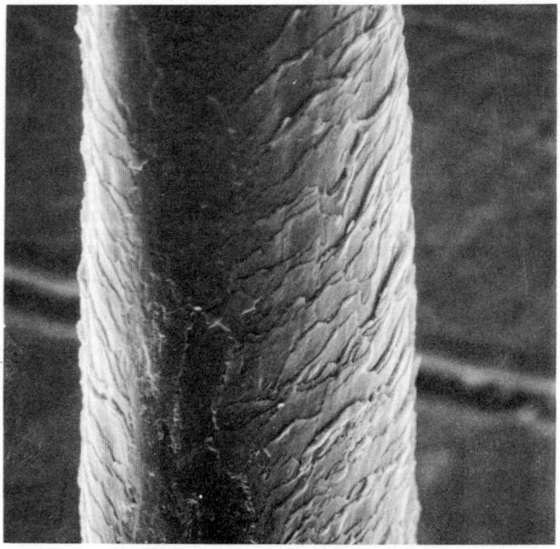

DAMAGED HAIRSHAFT

exposing the cortex and pitting the hair shaft.

Unfortunately you can't really replace lost moisture or repair damaged hair. Instead, you need a strategy to make your dried or even damaged hair look, feel, and behave more like the winner it once was.

A MIXED BAG

Don't be fooled into assuming you can escape dry-hair woes just because you happen to have an oily scalp. Home or work environments where heating and cooling systems deplete the air's moisture can be as hard on your hair as intensive competition in a club sports tournament, weekend frolics at the lake, or just lolling on a beach, with all the exposure to sun and wind. Any one of those settings, indoors or out, could produce the maddening combination of oily scalp with dry hair, vulnerable to all the pitfalls that accompany any other dry-hair dilemma. So you need a tricky strategy that will reduce your scalp oils yet moisturize your hair.

HAIR CARE'S CATCH-22

What's more, nature doesn't work alone. Many of your own efforts to get control of your hair are just as drying as the elements—especially if you believe, as some women seem to, that if it's worth doing, it's worth overdoing. For the equipment that helps you adjust nature's "errors" (like giving you straight hair when you would have preferred waves or making you a brunette when red hair would have pleased you much more) can work against you if used to excess.

Some of the adjustments you achieve—with *heated rollers* or a *blow-dryer,* for example—produce relatively short-term benefits. In these instances humidity is usually the culprit, forcing the hair shaft back to its natural wave pattern. So you use the appliances to coax it into a different shape. Other changes, accomplished with chemicals, such as *permanent waving lotions* or *hair-coloring agents,* last longer. But all changes—long-term or short-term—are attainable only by altering the shaft of hair in some way.

Chemicals lift the cuticle layer, increasing the hair shaft's porosity. That's how a coloring agent or waving lotion penetrates to the cortex to produce the shade or curl pattern you want. Also, thanks to the raised cuticles, your hair feels and looks fuller and fluffier, having acquired more body.

So much for the good news. The bad news is that with the cuticles raised, you're bound to lose shine. Also, the exposed cortex layer becomes more susceptible to drying. So you can see how overtreating may well leave you with extreme porosity and severe hair damage.

EMOTIONAL UPS AND DOWNS

And if all that weren't enough, other outside influences tend to compound the problem. Emotional stress, often resulting from women's changing roles over the past two or three decades, can be just as devastating to your hair as to other aspects of your well-being. Most dermatologists will tell you that the anxieties, conflicts, and tensions inherent in balancing careers outside the home with responsibilities to families and other components of a modern life-style have dramatically increased hair problems among women, which range from consistently dry, lifeless hair with splitting ends to thinning—even balding.

INNER STRENGTHS AND WEAKNESSES

Of course, not every obstacle to healthy, manageable hair launches its offense from outside your body. Hormonal changes, such as those that come with pregnancy and menopause, can affect your hair. Illnesses can make an impact. In fact, physicians sometimes use hair analysis to help diagnose diseases, deficiencies, and excesses. Elevated sodium deposits on the hair shaft, for instance, could mean that you excrete too much salt in your perspiration, perhaps leaving you deficient in salt.

But, then, remedies can be just as disruptive to hair as maladies. The incredible range of medications at our disposal—such as contraceptive pills, cortizone, anticoagulants, anticancer chemotherapies, thyroid hormones, and some antihypertensive medications—can have a number of effects, from simply making hair dull, lifeless, or unmanageable to inducing hair loss or encouraging hair growth—perhaps where you don't want it. In fact, Minoxidil, a drug originally developed for internal use against hypertension (high blood pressure) is being used successfully as a topical remedy against certain kinds of baldness; it has FDA approval for external use only in that connection.

Drugs can also influence how your hair takes to chemical treatments, like perming and coloring. I experienced this problem firsthand when a client who had been using one hair-coloring formula for more than five years wound up with a radically different shade in the touched-up areas closest to her scalp even though the colorist had applied the very same formula.

After we all had recovered from the shock, I asked my client about recent events or activities that might have accounted for the strange result. Eventually she mentioned a change in her medication sometime before—the probable cause, we later learned, of her hair's unusual interaction with the coloring agent.

Obviously, proper treatment for illness takes precedence over any cosmetic improvement. But even when you're ill, you can retain some control. If you develop a condition different from your previously normal state, whether it's an illness or a change like pregnancy or menopause, learn all you can about its implications, including how it might affect your hair. The same applies for drugs you may take and their potential side effects. And certainly discuss them, not only with your physician but also with your hairdresser. At the very least you may avoid unwelcome surprises. Perhaps your altered body chemistry won't change the way your touch-up or perm turns out. But wouldn't you rather find out with a simple strand test than by risking a disaster all over your head?

EXERCISING GREATER CONTROL

You also can strengthen the hair shaft's basic position by getting enough exercise. It may seem silly to raise this point in a book primarily aimed at active individuals. But if you limit your physical exertion to weekends or certain seasons, you may not be getting enough exercise. Shaping up, perhaps with a regular workout, can enhance your hair along with the rest of you.

Activities that bolster your general health have to be good for your hair. But their benefits to your attitude are just as important to your appearance. Few people I've ever met actually enjoy the strain and pain of stretching toward that last mile at the end of a day's run. But people who run, work out, or exercise regularly in some other way will tell you how great they feel about themselves simply for having done it.

Regular exercise often helps alleviate tensions that can harm your hair. And of course, exercise tends to improve your circulation. This benefit is vital to your hair because nutrients reach the root of the hair shaft through the bloodstream. Therefore, poor circulation impedes its nourishment. And undernourished hair can undermine your control.

THE PROOF IS IN THE EATING

Of course, even superb circulation won't help you much *if you don't get enough nutrients in the first place.* I'm talking about the foods you eat, not the foods you might want to smear or pour on your head. Now and then clients ask my opinion of certain "nourishing" kitchen remedies for problem hair they've read or heard about somewhere. I tell them what I'll tell you now: Nutrients nourish by ingestion, not by topical application.

Sure, a glob or two of mayonnaise (one ingredient commonly used) will help condition your hair. It contains oil, and almost anything oily will do the same. Beer, another mentioned often, will give your hair body. It contains sugar and other residue-forming ingredients that cling to the hair shaft. But it also can leave your hair smelling like a brewery.

So why not opt for the far more pleasant—and, I think, more beneficial—experience to be had with commercial products? They're formulated specifically to give you the results you want yet leave your hair looking, feeling, and smelling like fresh, clean hair—not like yesterday's lunch.

I'm not implying that kitchen remedies offer no major benefits to your hair. But you must eat or drink them to gain significantly from them! Mayonnaise, in fact, is one of several dependable sources of essential fatty acids. These nutrients are vital not only to your hair but to your overall well-being; they help transport other nutrients, via the bloodstream, all over your body for use in building cells.

Unfortunately health professionals tell us that our bodies can't produce enough of these essential fatty acids to sustain us. And with our current penchant for crash dieting—often avoiding fats entirely for protracted periods—deficiencies in these important nutrients may be more common than we realize. Among the possible results: problem skin, including scaly scalp (after all, what is your scalp if not an extension of your facial skin?) and thin, dull, lifeless hair.

So, if these conditions plague you, perhaps your diet is too low in fats. A tablespoon or two of salad oil added daily to a menu that has been lacking in fats just might help alleviate them. Many people make sure their pets regularly get a small amount of oil to help keep their coats shiny and healthy-looking. Shouldn't we do as much for our own hair?

Your best source of fatty acids is natural vegetable oils. Happily for cholesterol-watchers, some of these oils that are highest in polyunsaturated fats (the kind, such as corn and soybean oils, that help reduce cholesterol levels) also have the highest concentrations of fatty acids. Animal fats, such as cream, butter, egg yolks, and meat fats, contain the lowest percentages.

Another function of fats in the diet is to improve your ability to absorb other fat-soluble nutrients. One example is vitamin A. If you don't get enough, you could wind up with eyesight problems, skin disorders, including severe dandruff, and dry, lackluster hair. Your richest vitamin A sources are leafy vegetables like lettuce, spinach, and kale and other greens such as broccoli, string beans, and celery as well as carrots, yellow squash, sweet potatoes or yams, and apricots.

Protein, which, next to water, constitutes the largest percentage of your body, is vital to the structure, growth, and repair of all living cells. Without protein, there would be no life. Its specific benefits to hair become apparent when you realize that your hair, nails, skin, and muscle tissue are comprised almost entirely of protein. So you need this nutrient to keep your hair healthy, resilient, and manageable. And while studies show that protein added to hair care products can make hair feel and look thicker, topical applications are no substitute for protein provided by foods.

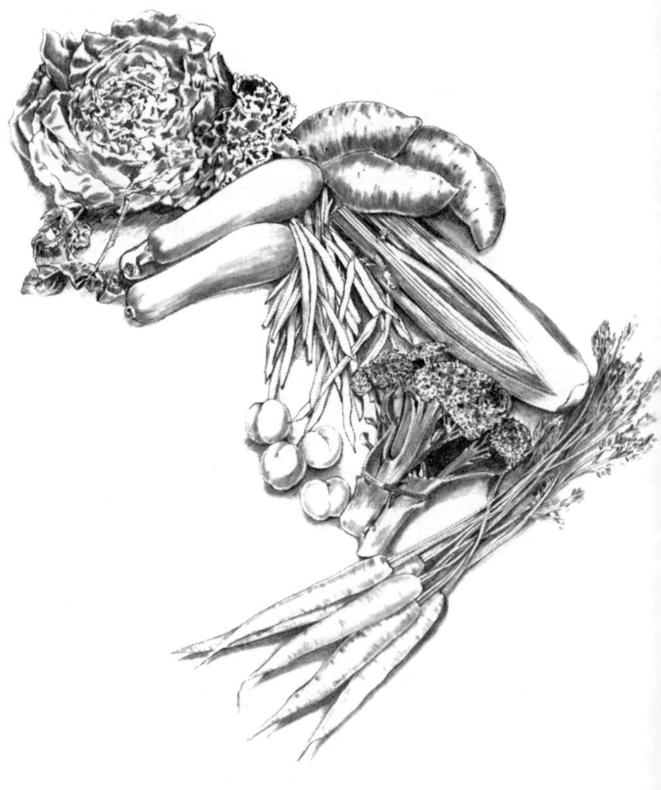

That is not to say that you must dig into a steak dinner several times a week. A very long list of protein sources aside from red meats includes fish, fowl, cheese, egg whites (yolks contain all the fat), milk, and a wide range of nuts, whole-grain foods (breads, cereals, pastas, etc.), peas, and beans.

I make a point of specifying only a few nutrients here because apart from their other functions, they offer particular benefits to your hair, your scalp, and the rest of your skin. Obviously you need the whole range of vitamins and minerals. In many cases, they're interdependent. Vitamin A, for example, needs zinc to metabolize within your system. The presence of vitamin D can make the difference between absorbing calcium and losing it.

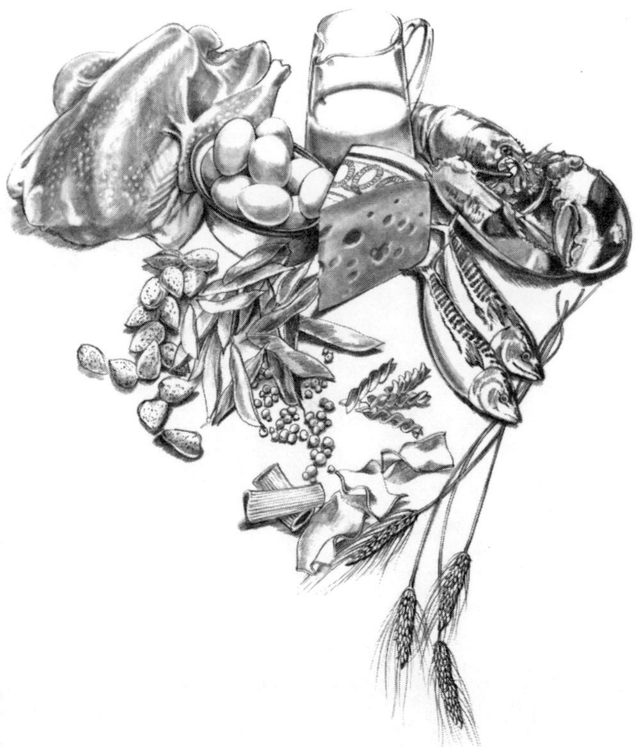

Should you therefore plunge into a program of megadose vitamin therapy? No. On the contrary, nutritionists emphasize that with an adequate, properly balanced diet, readily available to most of us within the ordinary range of foods at our disposal, we should have little need for supplements. Also, megadose vitamin therapy, without proper professional guidance, could backfire, possibly producing toxic reactions if you got too much of a vitamin that your body stores, such as A.

Still, supplements may be useful at certain times on the advice of a health professional who can prescribe suitable combinations and dosages if you need them. These could include B vitamins, especially if you're heavily into sports, because they are essential to your health and seem highly vulnerable to modern food-refining techniques that destroy nutrients.

Yet nutritionists report consistently better results with natural foods supplying the entire B complex than with synthetics. Many B vitamins occur together in foods like liver, brewer's yeast, whole-grain foods, vegetables such as beets, turnip greens, broccoli, kale, spinach, and watercress, and dairy products such as yogurt, which comes in low-fat and *non*fat forms and is among the best all-around nutritious foods.

What nutritionists are saying about a diet to promote good health applies to other aspects of your quest for beautiful, healthy hair: Your strongest offense is a good defense. And this book is about strategies to help you develop both.

THREE

IS YOUR HAIR READY TO WEAR?

Does your hair make you look and feel wonderful? Does it satisfy the demands of your busy schedule and stand up to high stress? Can you whip it into shape at a moment's notice for any occasion? A yes answer to all these questions describes what I call high performance hair. And high performance hair is almost always ready to wear.

To determine whether or not your hair has what it takes to perform well for you most of the time or where it falls short, answer the multiple-choice quiz below. Select one reply for each question, and allow five points for every question you answer with an (a), three points for every (b) response, and one point for every (c).

1. If you don't use a dryer after you shampoo your hair, does your hair dry in
   (*a*) ten to twenty minutes?
   (*b*) twenty to forty minutes?
   (*c*) more than forty minutes?
2. When your hair dries by itself, does it
   (*a*) give you a wash-and-wear look you love?
   (*b*) give you a wash-and-wear look that could use some extra attention?

(*c*) look washed but totally unwearable as is?

3. When you take the time to blow-dry and style your hair, do you usually spend
   (*a*) ten to fifteen minutes?
   (*b*) twenty to thirty minutes?
   (*c*) thirty-five minutes or longer?
4. Do the time and effort you initially invest with your dryer and styling brush usually leave you with hair that needs
   (*a*) no more than quick finishing touches with a brush or comb and a dash of hair spray?
   (*b*) spot touch-ups with a curling iron or a few heated rollers?
   (*c*) the time and attention it takes for an entire set?
5. Does the whole process usually produce
   (*a*) precisely the look you want?
   (*b*) not your favorite look but an acceptable hairstyle?
   (*c*) disappointing results?
6. During the course of the day does your hair require
   (*a*) little, if any, attention?
   (*b*) a quick brushup?
   (*c*) a fair amount of additional help from appliances?
7. When you're at the beach, do you
   (*a*) rinse the salt water out of your hair after every swim and apply a protective hairdressing?
   (*b*) keep your head covered?
   (*c*) ignore your hair entirely?
8. To keep your hair at high performance level, do you
   (*a*) find you can count on your hair's natural color and wave pattern?
   (*b*) need at least one chemical process (color or perm)?
   (*c*) need coloring *and* perming?
9. After an aerobic workout does your hair tend to
   (*a*) bounce back into shape?
   (*b*) perk up as soon as your perspiration dries?
   (*c*) droop hopelessly until you can rewash and restyle it?
10. Do those summer fun-in-the-sun weekends leave your hair
    (*a*) in almost capital condition with little, if any, extra attention?

(*b*) lacking some of its usual life and luster?
(*c*) suffering from the frizzies and split ends?

11. Do you need intense conditioning treatments
    (*a*) once or twice a month?
    (*b*) two to four times a month?
    (*c*) four to six times a month?
12. Do you keep your hair short because
    (*a*) you love the way you look in short hair?
    (*b*) it gives you wash-and-wearability you never got with longer hair?
    (*c*) the very thought of daily bouts with all that hair-tangling, nerve-jangling length turns you off every time you decide to let it grow?
13. Do you keep your hair long because
    (*a*) you look glamorous in long hair?
    (*b*) a ponytail is the only style that keeps your hair in place during your hectic day?
    (*c*) you don't know what else to do with it?
14. Does your haircut last
    (*a*) six to eight weeks?
    (*b*) four to six weeks?
    (*c*) two to four weeks?
15. For a last-minute invitation to a gala evening out, are you likely to
    (*a*) come up with a gala evening hairstyle within fifteen minutes?
    (*b*) easily reshape your daytime hairdo into a presentable evening look, given twenty to thirty minutes and the help of heated rollers?
    (*c*) have to start from scratch with a fresh shampoo for a stint of forty-five minutes or more?

If you've scored more than sixty-five points, congratulations! You must be doing something right. Read on to see how you can make your high performance hair perform even better.

A score between fifty and sixty-five isn't poor either. Though your hair needs help, you're on your way to getting the best those tresses can give you. Perhaps little more than a shift or two in the products you use to keep your hair in shape or a lesson in choosing and using the most efficient styling tools will push you over that finish line.

If you've scored below fifty points, number yourself among the have-nots—the vast majority. But don't despair. With a new approach to haircare and hairstyling, you, too, can develop what it takes to have high performance hair. In fact, you'd do well to develop a whole new way of looking at your hair in terms of what it can or can't do.

GO WITH WHAT YOU'VE GOT

Going with what you've got doesn't mean that if you feel stuck with what nature gave you, you must stay stuck. But it does mean you should compare the hair you have with the hair you've been trying to have. How radically different are they? How long, how hard, and how often do you have to struggle to keep yours that other way?

It would seem utterly ridiculous, for example, if bodybuilder Gladys Portugues, whom you may recall from the movie *Pumping Iron II,* were to try to make her thick, curly hair hang in one sleek length to her waist. Can it be done? Sure! Her hair is almost long enough (see photo on page 84). And everyone knows you can make curly hair straight and vice versa. But she'd have to stand for hours with a brush and blow-dryer, just stretching all that length—not her favorite way to work out her arms, I'd say.

For me, the notion is only a bit more ludicrous than a vision of you spending a half hour or so forcing your hair to submit to a shape it won't hold when confronted with its natural resistance and the most ordinary day-to-day stresses. Obviously Gladys didn't cut her curly hair to the quick for the sake of low maintenance. But she did find that layering, which uses her texture and curl pattern to advantage instead of fighting with it, allows her to have the length she wants in a way that works for her hair type.

By the same token, fine, straight hair runs you into a problem if you want a very curly look. Even if you do it with a perm (and you can't get much curlier than you can with a perm), as your hair grows the new, unpermed area collapses. So you no longer get volume where you need it most: at the crown. Instead, you wind up with a Bozo look: flat on top and bushy all around the sides and back. The upkeep to avoid that result would be hard on your hair as well as on your crammed schedule.

I'm not suggesting that you suffer in silence with your straight-as-sticks hair if you want a softer feeling around your face. But you should set a realistic objective—a goal that's easily attainable and maintainable with the hair you inherited. By all means, permanent-wave your hair—not so much to make it curly as to make it more manageable, so you can do more with it without becoming a slave to it.

Former Olympic skier Suzy Chaffee, whose fine, straight hair frustrated her both on and off the slopes, agreed to this approach and has never regretted it for a moment.

"I was always battling with my hair," Chaffee recalls. "You get to look pretty ratty out there. Skiers have to put up with those sweaty hats or with windy, cold weather. And from there it's downhill all the way for your hair, too, especially after that first run when the snow starts to fall."

The perm became our strategy to make Suzy's hair behave more like the ideal: medium-textured hair with a tendency to wave.

"Now I can be out all day, even get caught in a snowstorm, and my hair still looks good," she says.

Perhaps the most terrific feature of her perm is the versatility Suzy never would have enjoyed had she tried for a curly head. Because she chose to enhance her fine, straight hair rather than fight it, she now can set it on heated rollers for waves or soft curls, she can stretch it straight with a brush and blow-dryer, or she can combine the two techniques for a festive evening look. Any one of those approaches takes little effort and a minimal investment of Suzy's time.

What type of hair do *you* have, and how can you make it perform best for you? You've owned that head of hair long enough to know whether it's curly, wavy, straight, or somewhere in between. But since so many people tend to confuse texture with density and sparsity, here are a few guidelines for identifying your hair's texture. I'll also recommend the hairstyling approaches I think will give you gratifying results, with minimum fuss and maximum staying power, along with some of your best hair helpers, which will be spelled out in more detail in Chapter 5.

Is your hair superstraight, usually glossy and silky to the touch? Does it resist curling and then droop an hour or less after you have removed the rollers? Does it go limp in humid weather and get oily hours after you've shampooed, especially when you condition, too? If all or most of these characteristics describe your hair, it's *finely textured.*

Strive for hairstyles ranging from moderately wavy to the straighter, smoother looks your hair naturally assumes with some of the volume, lift, and staying power you never thought you could have. A perm may give you the wave or curl you crave, but it's not your only avenue to rewarding results.

Other hair helpers: mousses; gels; hair sprays; even hair-coloring agents if you plan to perk up your shade anyway. When matched with the right styling tools, they will give you varying degrees of extra body and control, depending on how submissive or stubborn your hair is.

Finely textured hair also comes in curly and wavy patterns. It often looks wispy, almost as if it were spun out of air, feels soft and delicate, and tends to resemble cotton candy in humid weather. You can achieve sleeker looks with the help of a blow-dryer and brush and a little patience, especially with all-one-length hair. But why spend fifteen minutes or more stretching your entire head of hair as straight as you can when you know those curls or waves will start to reappear before you get halfway through your day, especially in even slightly damp air? Hardly an economical use of your time, not to mention the frustration all that wasted effort generates.

Your more realistic objective is hairstyles ranging from curly to wavy, perhaps with some smoothness in places (such as at the temples or in the crown area) now and then for greater versatility.

Your potential hair helpers are mousses, gels, hairsprays, and, of course, the right styling tools, which will be discussed in considerable detail in Chapter 5. Here again, if you want to spruce up your hair color, your fine, wispy hair can benefit significantly from the extra body you get with hair-coloring agents.

Coarse hair, at the opposite end of the spectrum, feels thick and heavy, tends to lack luster, and puffs up and out when exposed to damp air. If it's wavy or curly, humidity makes it more so. But even in dry weather, coarse curls and waves stubbornly resist efforts to straighten them. So, like Gladys Portugues, you'd do well to save your precious time and energy for efforts that produce lasting rewards instead of wasting them on the constant struggle to keep your hair straight.

Certainly, chemical straightening makes almost as viable an option for you as permanent-waving does for other types of hair. But if your hair is curly to very curly, be prepared for regular stints at the hair salon. They may bog you down more than you realize—not quite in keeping with a quick and easy hair care philosophy.

I recommend, instead, that you opt for hair in curly or wavy styles—long or short. You can vary your style occasionally if you have the time to achieve a smooth look in certain areas, but I don't suggest doing that on a daily basis, especially if you shampoo often and have to get where you're going fast.

Coarse wavy hair, naturally, will give you somewhat more flexibility than coarse, curly hair, but even curly hair offers a sufficient number of styling options for variety.

Coarse, straight hair does especially well with geometric cuts, such as Dorothy Hamill's wedge, or all-one-length blunt-cut bobs.

Your best hair helpers whether your coarse hair is curly, wavy, or straight are gels (mousses are far too light to handle your resistant hair) and hair sprays (always with extra holding power) teamed with the styling tools to help you get the look you want quickly and efficiently.

Although regular hair conditioning is advisable for everyone, the right conditioners used with scrupulous regularity will significantly increase your hair's shine and manageability and decrease the amount of time you have to spend making it do whatever you want it to. A natural henna makes an excellent tinting choice for coarse hair, especially for black women since it not only enriches the natural shade without changing your hair color but also smooths the hair shaft, giving the hair more shine and manageability.

Medium-textured hair—the most manageable of the three textures—allows you to go curly, wavy, or straight with the least amount of resistance. It also tends to hold its temporary shape reasonably well until your next shampoo. But only wavy hair in this category is truly versatile, in that it usually can assume and hold a curled or straight pattern equally well. The hairstyles that give you the greatest handling ease depend on a broad spectrum of circumstances, including how your hair is cut and how it decides to behave on a given day. Humidity, for example, will make it wilt at times and puff out at other times. Although your hair may be somewhat unpredictable on occasion, medium-textured hair also gives you the greatest leeway. You have precisely the kind of hair everyone else wants.

If your medium-textured hair is straight, you should be able to get wonderful volume and lift in a variety of smooth or even wavy styles with relative ease. Save curlier looks, if you want to try them, for special occasions when you can make a point of setting aside extra grooming time.

Obviously those curly styles are your best option if your hair has a lot of curl. But you also can vary your hairstyle for smoother, wavy effects with relatively little effort.

Almost all the hair helpers I cite for the other hair types will give you even more control over your already relatively manageable hair. Which of them you use depends largely on the effects you're after as well as the shape and condition of your hair.

If you don't already have a preconceived idea of how you want to look, a little research may unearth several potential winning possibilities for you. Start by looking through this book, in which you'll find some of the best examples available anywhere of high performance women and their high performance looks. You can also thumb through sports magazines for photo features on celebrities you admire and through general-interest publications that run life-style articles on famous active women. Such an article includes photos, as a rule, and will give you insight into how the woman puts herself together during her leisure time.

The best test of a sportswoman's hairstyle is during tournament play and other events, for that's when you see the hair in action!

Obviously not every look you like will necessarily work for you. But even one that may not be quite right may have some feature that will work well within the context of your own style. In other words, adapt, don't copy! A little creativity and imagination can go a long way.

Your own distinctive style, for instance, might benefit from some of the subtle highlighting you see in roller skater April Allen's hair (see photo on page 69) but in a shorter haircut such as the one golf pro Muffin Spencer-Devlin wears (photos on pages 125–127). Or you may like the versatility of the longer layers in Martina Navratilova's haircut (see photo on page 72) with a curl pattern similar to Suzy Chaffee's permed hair.

How can you be sure a particular style or cut will work for your hair if you don't know what kind of hair your chosen role model has? In some cases you can tell just by the way the hair does or doesn't move with the player in motion—especially with the extreme hair types (fine and coarse). If you're not sure, however, clip a photo of the style you want and take it to your hairdresser. He or she should be able to advise you quickly whether or not the style makes sense for you or can be modified in some way to give you a similar look that's more manageable for your hair.

But ultimately *you* should be the one to combine a realistic appraisal of your hair's potential with the most efficient hair care and styling aids. With a little professional help now and then and almost no fuss on your part you'll have high performance hair that's almost always ready-to-wear.

FOUR

GET YOUR HAIR IN TOP FORM

I find it thoroughly exasperating that women who work hard to keep their bodies fit do little to enhance the condition of their hair. After all, isn't our hair part of our bodies? Shouldn't we want to keep it as fit as we keep our other parts?

Everyone wants healthy hair; healthy is better than unhealthy. Healthy hair provides the very foundation for what I call sportsworthy hairstyles, those that require minimum fuss yet make you look and feel sensational, even while you're moving at a frenetic pace. Only hair in top form will retain its elasticity—your key to the kind of control that will give you the gorgeous hairdos you want.

Your hair won't stay healthy all by itself any more than your body would stay in shape without some help. Believe me, keeping your hair in condition takes a lot less effort. Still, I find that all too many women neglect this facet of fitness simply by not using the right products for their specific hair care needs. Busy, active women seem the most cavalier in this respect.

When I began styling heads on the Ladies Professional Golf Association circuit, I quickly learned that these women tended to use the handiest grooming aids while on the road, giving no thought to any other criteria. More often than not, that meant grabbing whatever they happened to find in their hotel rooms. What could be more convenient? No need to stop and shop for shampoo when hotels provide it as a courtesy.

Never mind that the shampoos in those cute little sample packages are usually for normal hair, and "normal" rarely describes an athlete's hair. So what if all the sun and sweat, especially during tournaments, frizzes the fluff and wilts the waves, not to mention numerous other hair problems common to the sporting life? Do women notice the effects of the elements on permed and color-treated hair or realize that frequent washing, running for trains and planes, or other stresses inherent in competition take a toll on hair and scalp?

Certainly my clients (even those who once were unmindful of hair care) seek ways to cope with such issues. Most work for hours on end, day in and day out, in environments controlled by heating or cooling systems that deplete the air's moisture. Many also indulge in pastimes that repeatedly expose them to sun, wind, and other harsh elements. And you do likewise if you support your Little Leaguer by yelling yourself hoarse from those sun-drenched bleachers or get out often to root for a local football team on nippy afternoons. Do you enjoy brisk walks through the park, bicycling around your neighborhood, joining family and friends for barbecues, marshmallow roasts, and other similar outings? These outdoor activities, and others like them, can make you vulnerable to nature's elements, which compound the drying effects of the indoors environments we create for ourselves. Both tend to rob your hair of moisture, producing those awful symptoms of damaged hair: dull, dry, brittle, and highly porous hair that has no elasticity, tends to split at the ends, and won't do a thing you want it to.

Active individuals also have to deal with the effects of salt, especially during warm-weather months. Whether it comes from your perspiration, from the water you swim in, or from both, salt is drying and as harsh to porous hair as to any open wound. A hat that blocks the rays on a sunny beach may protect your face, but it can harm your hair unless it offers good ventilation (as in a straw chapeau) so that air can circulate. Without the benefit of quick evaporation, the salty perspiration from your scalp will descend on your hair and start ravaging it.

Swimming in chlorinated water can be equally damaging—actually worse if your hair is tinted, permed, straightened, or chemically treated in any way. Chlorine is a bleach, bound to lighten treated hair somewhat. But the greatest impact comes from copper compounds in chemicals added to retard algae growth and from the pool's pipes, usually made of copper (which turns green all by itself on oxidation). The combination can work a green cast into your hair color.

Beyond that, anyone who swims regularly faces the constant chore of detangling wet hair. This produces yet another kind of "tress stress."

And what about the frustrations you feel when your hair gets zapped repeatedly with humidity on all those not so lazy but decidedly hazy days of summer because that's when you spend so much more time outdoors? No matter that you, your dryer, and your styling brush invest considerable teamwork daily to stretch your curly hair smooth. Within minutes after you have ventured out, it starts to form ringlets, puff up and out, even frizz. Or maybe your straight-as-sticks hair, which begins most days in soft waves with the help of heated rollers, droops in damp weather along with that high you always get from just knowing how superb you look. Even in-between hair won't hold a style that deviates from its normal curl or wave pattern in high humidity. If only those lovely, low-humidity days weren't so few and far between. Right?

Well, yes and no! Remember, dry air—supportive though it may be to your hairdo—plays havoc with your hair by depriving it of the moisture it needs. Humidity, which clearly undermines your styling efforts, does so because your hair tends to grab moisture right out of the air—like water rushing in to fill a sponge. If these simple facts of life seem like a classic no-win situation, cheer up. While neither you nor I can do much to influence the weather or the air around us at work, you can modify your hair's reaction to it. In this chapter I'll tell you how as well as how to handle some of the other occupational and recreational hazards to hair wrought by the way you live.

GIVE YOUR HAIR A SPORTING CHANCE: SHAMPOOS

You'd do well to learn one of the first lessons I teach all my clients: You can't just dump any old shampoo on your hair no matter what kind you have, what condition it's in, or which of many potential stresses you expose it to.

That is not to say most of the four hundred or so products on the market won't make your hair clean and fluffy; they will—temporarily at least—just by removing dirt and oil. But these days shampoos are formulated to help minimize common hair problems while they clean, giving your hair a considerable edge. So why not make the most of this advantage and ferret out the shampoo that will work hardest to lower your hair's handicap?

The differences essentially lie in the amount of oil and other moisturizers shampoos contain in proportion to their detergents, the primary cleaning agent in most shampoos. And the ratio of moisturizer to detergent you want depends largely on the condition of your hair and scalp. With oily hair and scalp you need less moisturizer and more cleansing agent to remove the excess oils. And that basically is what you get in a product labeled "for oily hair." Shampoos for dry hair, which needs extra moisturizing help, have the opposite formulation. More even distributions of moisturizer and cleansing agent give us shampoos for normal hair, which strikes the best balance between oiliness and dryness.

But—and I can't say this often enough—"normal" hair simply *isn't the norm* for active individuals. On the contrary, many have to wrestle with extremes of both oiliness and dryness.

Some of my clients have tried to tackle the combination of oily scalp and dry hair with shampoos that condition as they clean. Unsuccessfully, I might add. Certainly, conditioning shampoos can be a plus for hair repeatedly doused with scorching sun, searing winds, discoloring chlorine, or harsh salts. And without a doubt they offer a timesaving feature obvious in one-step washing and conditioning. But condition-while-you-wash shampoos also contain the highest concentrations of oil and other moisturizers that make an oily scalp even oilier. So they are not your best choice for dry hair if your scalp secretes too much oil for your hair to handle in the first place.

Instead, you want a shampoo for oily hair that will work harder to remove those scalp oils. After all, cleaning your scalp is a major objective of shampooing. Let your conditioner handle your dry hair dilemma.

Is your hair permed, straightened, or colored? Even if you've always had normal hair, once you treat it with any chemical that induces change your hair can't really qualify as normal. Chemicals dry hair and increase its porosity. Add nature's constant assaults on your head and other stresses that tend to deplete moisture, and you compound the hazards, making your hair vulnerable to all sorts of foul play. So, normal though it once was, your treated hair now probably needs special attention, including, among other things, a shampoo for chemically treated or just plain dry hair—unless you have an excessively oily scalp.

Clearly there is no reasonable way for me here to suggest specific remedies that will handle everyone's hair care needs. With so many shampoos and conditioners on the market and dozens of variables that could make one more effective than another, I can offer only guidelines.

You know whether your scalp is mostly dry, oily, or normal. With that knowledge and some attention to how your hair responds to the various stresses your life-style subjects it to, you have only to scan a few labels to find one or two shampoos that provide the kind of help it needs.

I like hair care products that contain botanical ingredients—the essences and extracts of herbs and other plant life that, although popular in cosmetics today, aren't exactly new to personal care. Evidence uncovered at one Neanderthal burial site suggests that we've valued plants for their curative and restorative powers almost since humankind first appeared on earth. From then on, plants flourished as soothers and healers, not only among a few clustered cultures but all over the globe.

Throughout history people have also found cosmetic uses for plants and their by-products. Eyeliners that adorned the lids of both men and women of ancient civilizations often came from almonds burned and crushed to make the gray and black powders called kohl. Almond, along with other plants such as jojoba, also provided oil to smooth and soften the skin. Throughout the ages people have cleaned and, in other ways, treated or pampered their hair and scalps with the likes of rosemary, nettle, yucca, and yarrow. And your herb-scented bath, so soothing to body and soul, is no modern innovation. Early Romans, Greeks, and Egyptians dunked mint, thyme, chamomile, juniper, pine, and endless other herbs and blossoms in their baths not only as relaxants or pick-me-ups but for the seductive powers attributed to their fragrances. That champion seductress of all time, Cleopatra, was said to have drenched her body and her barge with the scent of roses for a greater advantage in seducing Marc Antony.

Passage of time has done little, if anything, to diminish faith in the healing and enhancing properties of plants. The great

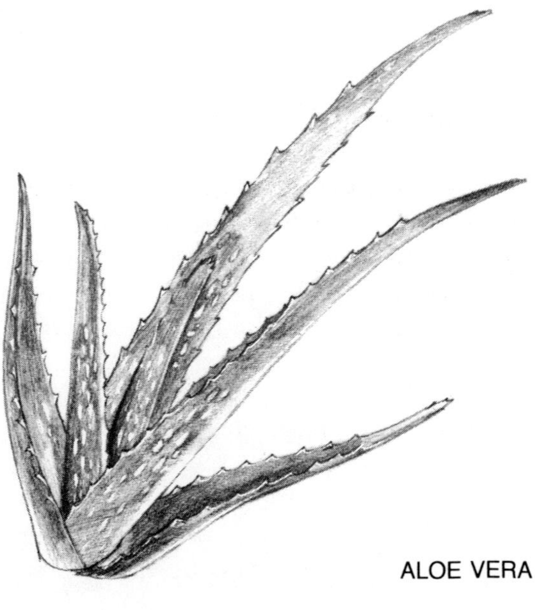

ALOE VERA

European manor houses of the Middle Ages came equipped with their own herb gardens, from which plants were plucked as needed for medicines and beauty potions. These days you might maintain an herb garden more for pleasure than practicality.

Major producers of beauty aids have found ways to harvest extracts and duplicate the essences of plants, which they use in today's highly sophisticated formulas.

Each is reputed to offer certain specific benefits. The extent to which botanicals impart benefits in modern hair preparations more than likely depends on your hair and on the nature and amount of the ingredient a particular product contains. At the very least they smell and feel wonderful for a luxurious and pampering effect—reason enough, in my opinion, to use them. Some of the more popular ingredients include:

Aloe vera, the sap (or juice as it's called, because of its high water content) from the aloe plant, is a well-established skin moisturizer, softener, smoother, soother, and healer, often found effective against burns and long recognized for its benefits to hair and scalp. For centuries among various cultures the sap straight from the plant was both shampoo and conditioner.

Chamomile, also found today in many skin care products, is the source of chamomile tea, an age-old remedy for everything from assorted internal disorders to jangled nerves. The fragrant yellow flower of this plant, a favorite for aromatic baths, yields a yellow coloring once used for

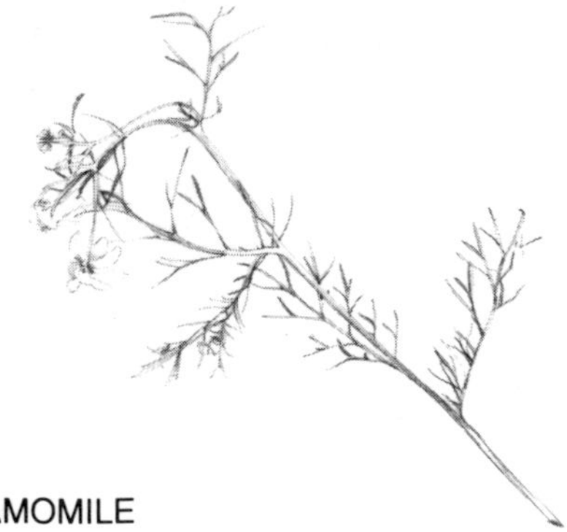

CHAMOMILE

blonding hair. Although modern blonding techniques certainly surpass its intensity and staying power, we still benefit from the color-enhancing properties of chamomile, which, in some hair products, puts sunny lights into blond or light brown hair.

Henna, from the leaves of the henna tree, is perhaps the best-known botanical source of coloring for the hair and other bodily adornments. Its popular cosmetic use dates from earliest recorded history to its current cosmetic and protective role in hair tinting.

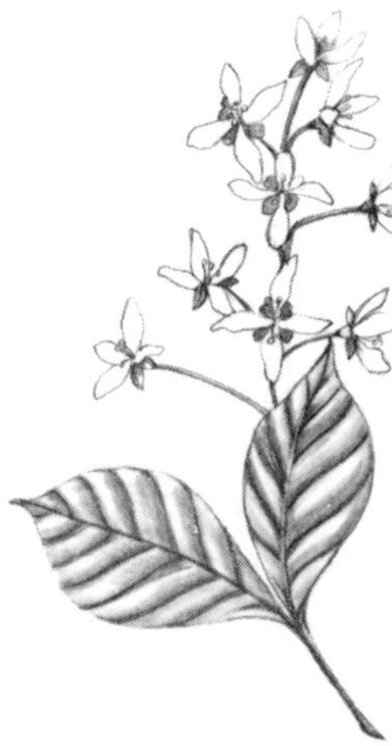

HENNA

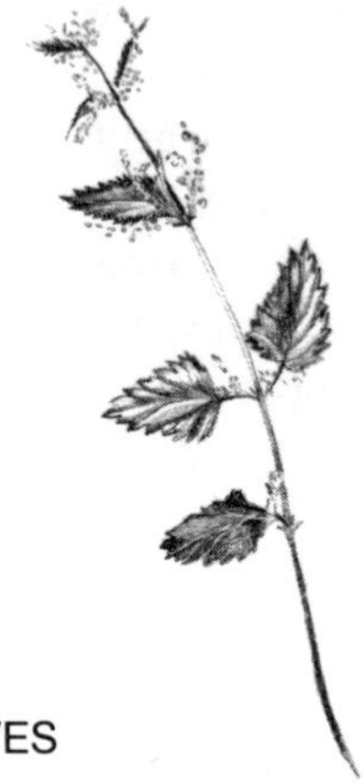

NETTLE LEAVES

Nettle leaves, used as a rub, have been credited with stimulating circulation. They've also been said to encourage hair growth, or at least to retard hair loss, when steeped in alcohol. Whether or not those hair tonics actually influence hair growth or loss, good circulation has been long recognized to promote healthy hair and scalp. In modern hair preparations the invigorating effects of nettle also tend to reduce oiliness.

Oats are the basis for the nonalkaline, mild oatmeal soaps and other similar preparations recommended from time to time by dermatologists for sensitive or troubled skin. In the seventeenth century the gentleness of oatmeal was much appreciated as a skin cleanser and a treatment to keep hands fashionably delicate-looking and wrinkle-free.

With delicateness decidedly out these days (especially in the sporting arena) shampoos and conditioners formulated with oats are valued for their gentle handling of hair and scalp. In that context

OATS

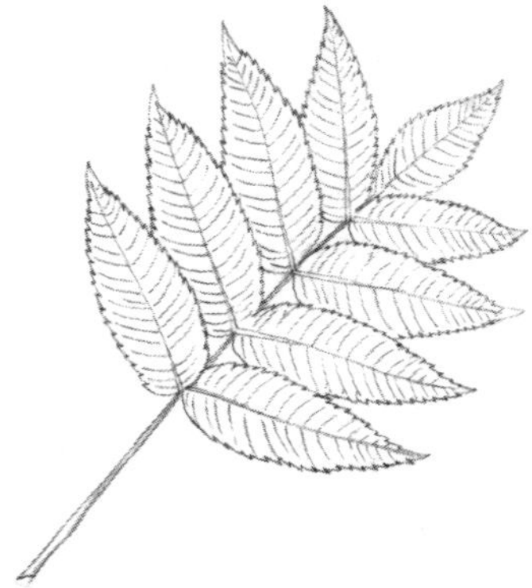

WALNUT LEAVES

they may score extra points with you if you shampoo as often as twice a day.

Oils of **jojoba, mink** (not a botanical but certainly natural), and **safflower,** as well as **glycerin** (a syrupy liquid extracted from animal and vegetable oils), are added to hair products for their ability to impart shine and draw moisture from outside sources or to hold it—all obvious benefits to most hair.

Walnut leaves and **parts of the walnut** itself yield several components often found to be soothing and healing. The leaves, which produce an herbal astringent, have been used in compresses as an antiperspirant and, in a variety of ways, for their anti-inflammatory effect against certain skin disorders. At one time they also were valued, along with the shell and other parts of the nut, for the brown liquid they make, which was commonly used to color hair. Today we don't rely on walnut leaves for hair tints any more than we depend on chamomile. But extracts from the plant exist in shampoos and conditioners as color enhancers for dark hair, while their astringent aspects may benefit a too oily scalp.

These do not represent all or even most of the botanical essences and extracts that may be found in today's hair preparations. But they're among the most popular ones you'll see in products sold at almost any outlet that carries beauty aids, starting from moderately priced shampoos at your local five-and-dime or discount store, to the mid-range groups distributed chiefly through department stores, right on up to the luxury lines available exclusively through your hair salon. They show up not only in shampoos but in other hair products—most notably, hair conditioners.

CONDITIONERS

I'm often asked, "If I use the right shampoo, is conditioning really all that important?" It usually means the client wants to cut corners whenever and wherever she can.

By now it must be pretty clear that no one could be more anxious than I am to save you time and help you eliminate unnecessary moves in your quest for beautiful hair. But cutting corners? That's another matter entirely, especially if you hope to eliminate conditioners in the process—a definite no-no, in my view. Remember, only healthy, manageable hair will give you the elasticity and control you need to make it do what you want when you want quickly and easily. And no matter what shampoo you use, conditioners are crucial to keeping your hair in top form. The more active you are, and the more time you spend outdoors, in any season, the more your hair needs their help.

I'm not suggesting that conditioners will repair damaged hair. Once hair is damaged, it's damaged! But they do fill the pores and smooth the cuticles on damaged hair or on any hair subjected to ordinary combing, shampooing, and other normal stresses. With both actions a conditioner, like the hair's original protective coating, smooths the hair shaft and helps retain moisture. Conditioners stand in for nature's depleted conditioning agents to make hair that's been around and abused for a while look and feel more like the newer, healthier hair growth closer to your scalp. As a result, the older hair behaves more as it did when it had all its elasticity.

Even in high humidity areas, where your hair gets moisture from the air by itself, it's a mistake to ignore conditioners when you're active and spend lots of time outdoors. In fact, you probably need them more, if only for the sake of your hairdo, according to golf pro Nancy Lopez. She should know. As a frequent winner on the LPGA tour Nancy spends a significant portion of her life outdoors. But only part of that is in pursuit of her golf earnings. During her days off you may well find Nancy out there in the stands cheering on her husband, Ray Knight, who plays third base for the New York Mets.

"I always condition after every shampoo, even in humid weather," Lopez says. "My hair simply doesn't seem to absorb the moisture it would otherwise."

As you have undoubtedly experienced, curly hair gets curlier in humid weather no matter how hard you worked to stretch it, and straight hair goes limp even though you curled it. This happens because temporary changes in the hair shaft, induced by the moisture it absorbs, force the hair to revert to its natural pattern. Also, humid weather expands the hair shaft and lifts the cuticle layer, encouraging that rough look we call the frizzies. Thanks to both effects, you wind up with either straight frizz or curly frizz. But conditioning enables you to control the extent to which your hair responds to humid weather because the process smooths and strengthens the hair shaft, making it more resistant to the effects of dampness.

Would any old conditioner give you that kind of control? Not really. For one thing, conditioners come in two basic categories: *instant conditioners and crème rinses,* which get rinsed out seconds after you apply them, and *intense conditioning treatments,* which remain on the hair anywhere from one minute to a half hour, depending on the product. You need both, though not at the same time, because although they appear to do the same job, they really serve two different purposes.

Instant conditioners and *crème rinses,* lighter than intense conditioning treatments, don't stay put long enough to penetrate the hair shaft. But they do provide quick, short-term benefits right at the surface by smoothing that hair and helping detangle it—reason enough, I think, to use one every time you shampoo, especially if you swim often.

Your hair is most fragile when it's wet, no matter what kind or how much of it you have. The very same moisture-induced changes that force your hair back to its natural wave pattern in high humidity also cause hair to go limp and stretch when it gets soaked. Consequently, wet hair loses some of its density and elasticity. And in that fragile state, without the detangling assistance you get from instant conditioners, ordinary combing can snap off hair shafts more readily.

Intense conditioning treatments, which also detangle hair, are a relatively easy way to rescue hair under lots of stress. They come in both crème and hot-oil formulas, heavier and thicker than instant conditioners because they have to cling long enough to penetrate the hair shaft. They usually contain more protein than instant conditioners, which adds to their longer-term benefits.

Obviously, hot-oil treatments, by definition, need heat to do their job, but I also recommend applying heat with the crème formulas to open those cuticles and pores for maximum penetration before the smoothing and closing action takes effect. Why not treat your hair to intense conditioning while you pamper your body in a sauna? Then you get two benefits in the time you spend for one.

It's a bit difficult to pinpoint just how often you need intense conditioning treatments since unlike instant conditioners and créme rinses, they're generally too heavy for use with every shampoo. You might require intense conditioning anywhere from two to four times a month or more often at certain times. The state of your hair, and, therefore, the kind of attention it needs, vary with climate, the nature and extent of your activities, and many other circumstances. If you play tennis indoors all winter, your hair may accumulate more oils from your scalp than during warm weather, when that bubble comes off the court, subjecting your hair to the vagaries of the outdoors. So you may have to condition less often in winter than in summer. On the other hand, if you ski bareheaded all winter and just lie around in a shady hammock in summer, the opposite could apply. Judicious use of intense conditioning treatments to mesh with your activities and keep up with your pace—along with an instant conditioner after every shampoo—can give you great control over your hair despite the pitfalls of a life-style that has you coming and going a lot more than it has you lying around in any season.

Suppose your hair goes limp and gets oily too fast from so much conditioning? Both problems can occur for a number of reasons: You may be using too much, or you may not be rinsing well enough. Or perhaps you condition your scalp along with your hair when in fact, you should keep conditioners off your scalp. Apply the product from your palms and fingers, not from the bottle, and with your head bent downward, first to the ends of your hair, which need it most. Then work it in gently, partway up toward the scalp, but not to it; the still healthy, newer hair growth closest to your scalp can do without conditioning until it has put up with the rigors of your life-style a bit longer.

Of course, it won't help much to apply conditioners properly if you're using the wrong ones. Each of the two basic categories—instant and intense—offers different levels of conditioning power, with products labeled accordingly. Some with higher moisturizer content, for example, advertise the "extra protection" you might need for coarse hair or during high-stress seasons. Others may boast special benefits to "extra-dry" hair that could describe your problem only during periods of concentrated exposure to sun.

"Extra-body" formulas, on the other hand, contain lighter moisturizing agents than the more powerful or standard formulas do, and they rinse out more readily. So, fine hair that tends to droop and accumulate oil quickly needs a lighter conditioning action. Also, the astringent properties of walnut and nettle leaves could make them your best botanical choices.

If you still can't get rid of those "greasies," don't abandon conditioners. Instead, apply them first; then shampoo—only once. Your hair will retain the benefits of conditioning yet lose a lot of its tendency to go limp and get oily quickly.

You can make conditioners a tool to help you gain control over your hair if you first choose the most efficient shampoo to minimize the problems that plague your hair and scalp and then determine which conditioners will cope best with stresses that confront your hair at any given time.

Then, by all means, go back to grabbing the handiest hair products, confident of keeping your hair in top form. Presumably your handiest hair care aids, from now on, will also be your best ones.

FIVE

PRO TOOLS AND HOW TO MASTER THEM

When clients tell me how they want their hair to look, whatever else they may describe, inevitably they get around to mentioning two elements: the soft fullness and the gentle upward curve you get with *volume* and *lift.* And it's no surprise. These are key ingredients for almost any successful hairstyle: volume because it imparts the look of rich, full-bodied, healthy hair and lift because we tend to perceive virtually everything uplifting in a positive light, especially when it relates to how we look.

You tone your body to keep muscles firm and uplifted. You apply makeup with an upward sweep for its most flattering effects. Even uplifting experiences have psychological benefits that tend to enhance your appearance. It follows that you want your hairstyle to do likewise by further emphasizing that upward illusion.

You know your hair can have that look. Your hairdresser has achieved it for you many times. Now, if only you could do the same and maintain it on your own . . . But how can you hope to get such results when even your hairdresser gives your hair more time and attention than you could dream of spending on it?

Believe it or not, you can! To make that wish come true, you have to control your hair. And to gain control, you need to do three things: Learn which among the sea of professional tools, appliances, and other styling aids available will make your hair do what you want it to with minimum fuss; develop a knack for using them; and turn that knack into a daily habit. Once you've accomplished the first two steps, you'll find those skills so indispensable that the third step will follow automatically. In this chapter I'll help you strive for that goal.

First, you should understand that for every styling effect you can create there are perhaps a dozen different ways to create it. And none of them is written in stone. In other words, *your* best path to the end result you want depends on your hair and which of the appropriate tools and styling aids you can use most comfortably and competently.

To help you select your optimum tools, I'll describe those I consider most useful, not only because they'll accomplish your goals but because once you've mastered the right implements for you, they'll keep your hairstyling routine uncomplicated. And simplicity is the key to giving you the control that will get you away from the mirror—fast! The right styling tools can help you use your grooming time economically so, even in the morning rush to shower, dress, and leave the house, you can get quick yet highly pleasing results.

BRUSHES

PLASTIC-QUILL BRUSH:

You'll probably use this one eighty-five percent of the time. It has flexible plastic quills set widely apart. And it's the *only* brush to use when your hair is wet. Your hair is weakest when wet, so using an instant conditioner isn't quite enough. You also need the firm but gentle action of those widely spaced quills that are pliable enough to give when you tug at a tangle. An ordinary brush with bristles set closely together can't slide through the weakened hair gently enough to detangle without damaging.

Your plastic-quill brush also will help you blow-dry your hair quickly since it doesn't retain water the way bristle brushes do. And it becomes a convenient styling tool, as I'll describe later in this chapter.

PADDLE BRUSH:

A blend of natural and synthetic bristles spaced closely together makes this brush good for the general tidying of dry hair only, for spreading scalp oils through your hair to increase its luster, for smoothing as the final step after styling, and for sprucing up a hairdo later.

SMALL PADDLE BRUSH:

This one can do all the things its larger version can when you're out and about.

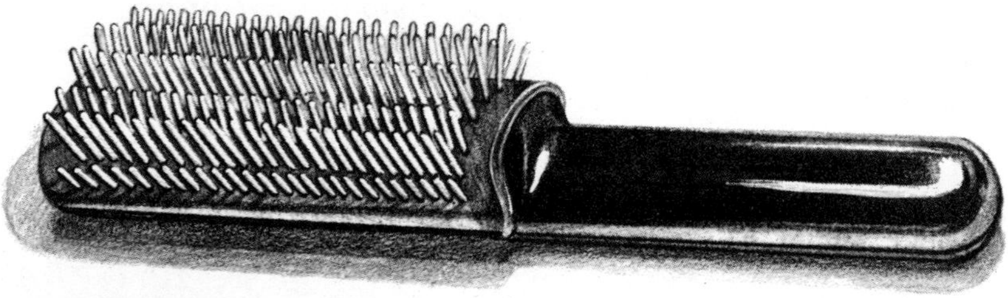

PLASTIC-QUILL BRUSH

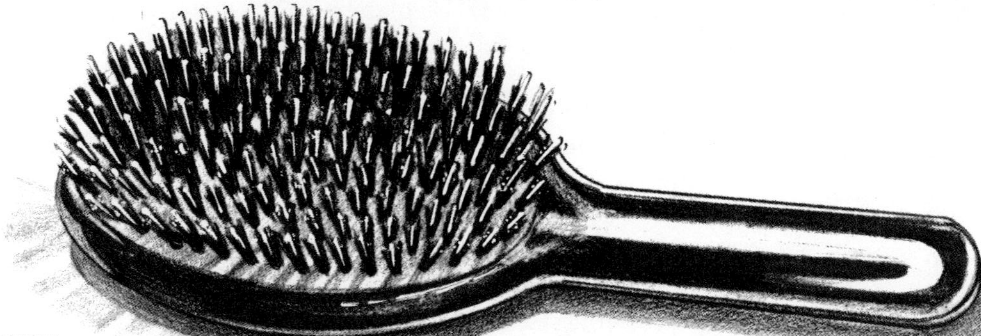

PADDLE BRUSH

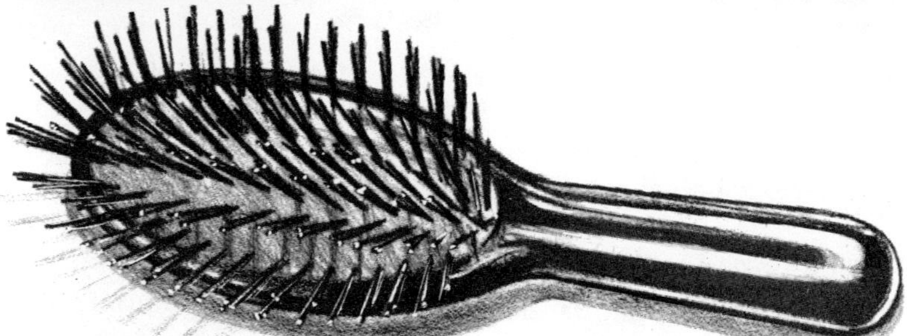

SMALL PADDLE BRUSH

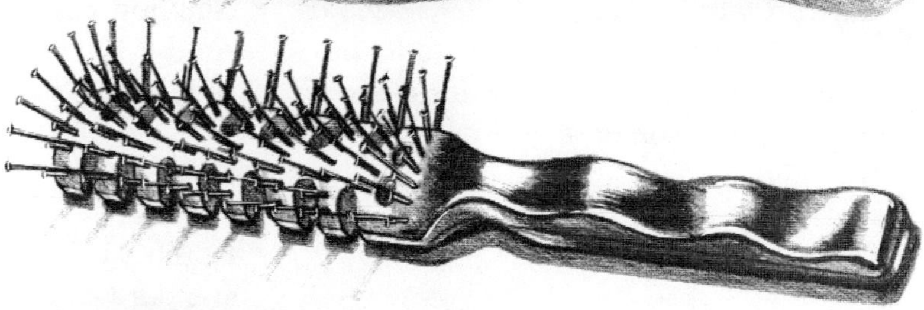

VENTED BRUSH

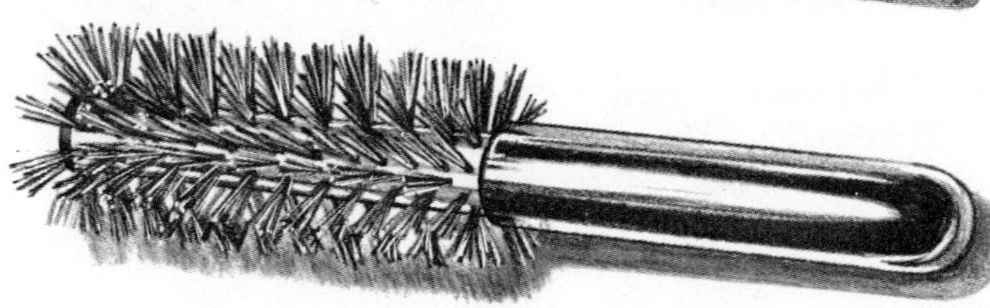

ROUND BRUSH

But I also like it for backbrushing to get volume (not to be confused with teasing).

VENTED BRUSH:

Its vented base and long plastic teeth, set in alternating rows of two lengths, helps speed drying thick, coarse, and curly hair. Therefore, the vented brush can be used for combing through wet hair if the hair is short and has coarse to medium texture. This brush is also an excellent finishing tool for any short or layered hairstyle.

ROUND BRUSH:

When used with a blow-dryer, this styling tool bends and curls the hair or stretches and smooths it, depending on the effect you want, which size you use, and how you use it. You can almost think of it as a roller since it performs a similar function. And like a roller, it comes in several diameters.

The brushes described here have specific functions. That is not to say you should run out and buy all five. Instead, consult the chart on page 52 for guidelines on which combination of brushes is most useful for your hair type and cut.

COMBS

In my experience, combs—even the few I describe below—have limited use. I especially don't like them for combing through the hair; the paddle brushes (large and small) do a better job. Still, certain combs can fit comfortably into a hairstyling routine. They include:

WIDE-TOOTH COMB:

This type is a reasonable alternative to the plastic-quill brush for detangling wet hair. Because its teeth are thick, blunt, and spaced widely apart, they are less likely than most other implements to damage wet hair. Keep in mind, however, that unlike the plastic quills, which are flexible, the teeth are rigid and won't give when they catch a snarl.

TAIL COMB:

This is a versatile tool for backcombing (again, not to be confused with teasing). The tail end is excellent for sectioning, parting, and lifting.

PICK:

Its widely spaced long teeth perform a function similar to the tail end of the tail comb. But they cover a wider area—a timesaving factor.

PICK-COMB:

I prefer this combination of a pick and a standard comb. Its variegated teeth on one end and long steel pins spaced widely apart on the other cut down on time by allowing you to section, part, lift, blend, and smooth quickly—all with the one instrument.

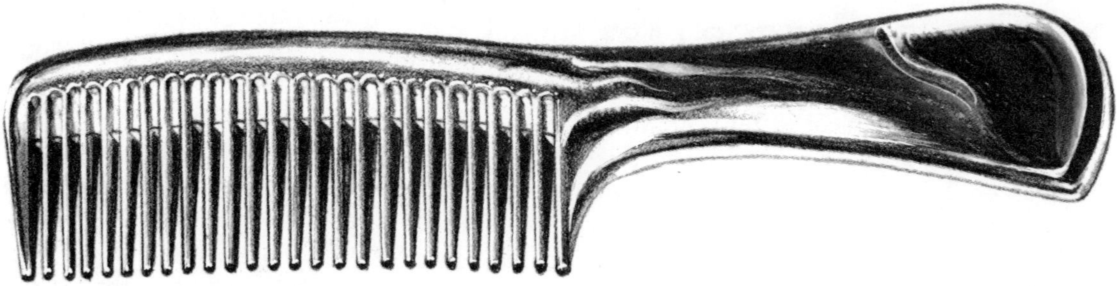

WIDE-TOOTH COMB

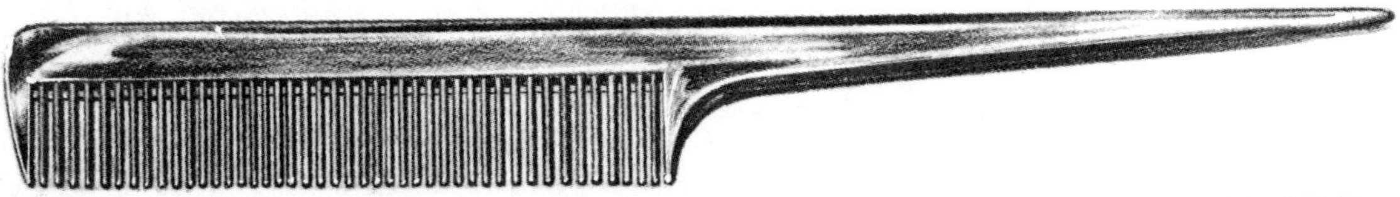

TAIL COMB

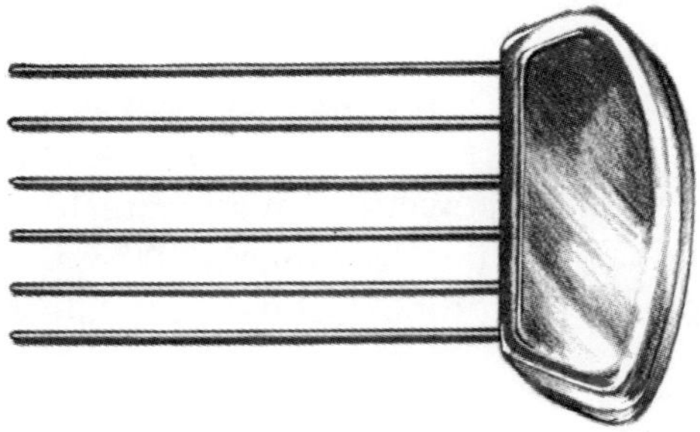

PICK

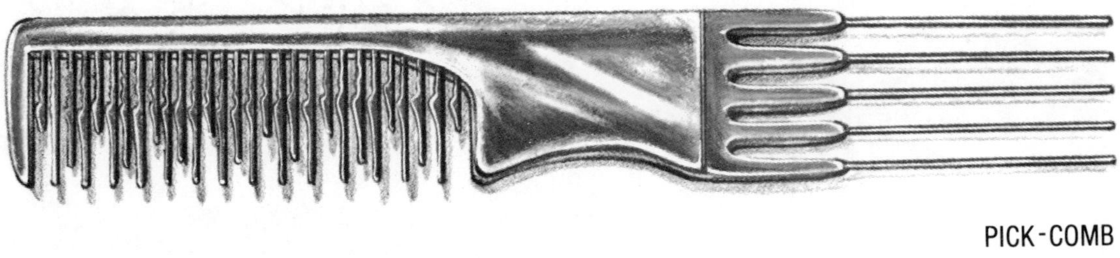

PICK-COMB

SAVING THE BEST FOR LAST

I now come to what could be your most useful combing-styling tool: *your fingers!* In a pinch—or even as a preference—you can use them effectively for everything from simple detangling and blow-drying to quickly executing a variety of intricate styling maneuvers, which I'll cover in the section on handling tools and appliances.

APPLIANCES AND OTHER IMPLEMENTS

BLOW-DRYERS:

If you're using an old 900-watt purse-size number, pitch it into the nearest trash can. I mean, you can't even dry your socks with that! I like a 1,500-watt dryer because it has lots of power that works quickly. Certainly, nothing less than 1,100 watts will do. Your optimum choice: a professional type 1,500-watt "gun" designed for consumer use and readily available at reasonable cost.

A standard attachment with most dryers is the concentrated hot-air nozzle. My advice: Scratch it! Concentrated heat damages or weakens the hair.

Use common sense in handling your dryer. Always read manufacturers' directions before using any appliance. Make sure the nozzle stays on course. If your curtains rustle and the window is closed, you may be drying those, but you're not drying your hair. Hold the dryer close enough to your head to be effective—about five or six inches away. But if your hand feels uncomfortably hot, the unit is probably too close, and you may be drying *out* your hair rather than drying it.

BLOW-DRYER DIFFUSER ATTACHMENT:

Available as a separate appliance, it diminishes the force of air by spreading it over a wider area. Of course, this slows the drying. But it's great if you have a natural

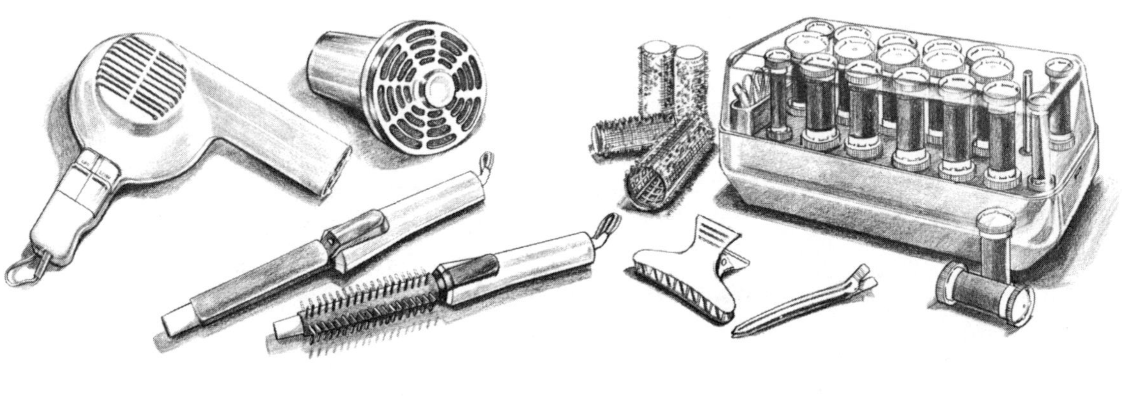

wave or curl you want to keep because the hair gets blown around a lot less. Therefore, you make up lost drying time by not having to invest much styling time—thanks to your hair's natural bend.

INSTANT HAIR SETTERS (HOT ROLLERS):

Some come with tiny teeth or ridges, which may or may not grip the hair better than smooth ones, making it easier to roll. However, they can get caught in your hair, especially if it's dry and porous. Smooth-surfaced rollers covered in velvet, on the other hand, prevent tangles and pulls, protect the hair from extreme heat, and curl just as effectively. I especially like the ones from Clairol that feature an inner core filled with wax providing gentle, longer-lasting heat and, therefore, longer-lasting curl.

CURLING IRONS:

These provide the fastest way to make a curl because you roll the iron in, take it out immediately, and *voilà!* you have a curl, whereas hot rollers have to stay in your hair for a few minutes. The type I like best for home use has a spring clip and a nonheating tip for easier handling.

HEATED STYLING BRUSHES:

A wand resembling a curling iron but with pliable, nonheating Teflon bristles that gently penetrate the hair, allowing contact with the heat from the wand.

VELCRO ROLLERS:

Not an electric appliance, they need other heat sources (blow-dryer, hood-dryer, etc.) or can be used while air-drying a set if you have at-home chores to do. Obviously they're not convenient in the same sense as hot rollers. Still, they're worth noting because the Velcro clings to the hair, making the rollers exceptionally easy to roll.

CLAMPS AND CLIPS:

These aid in sectioning hair for styling ease. They hold one area aside so you can work freely with another.

COMBING THROUGH WET HAIR

When you pop out of the shower, are you likely to grab the nearest comb or brush and tear it through your wet hair, beginning at the top? Don't do it! Those strands are weakest when they're wet. And it shouldn't surprise you that your crown is more susceptible to hair damage from all that pulling and tugging than any other part of your head. Moreover, participating in a sport that often has you out in the sun, the wind, and perhaps other harsh elements only compounds the problem.

Since damaged hair is harder to handle and needs more attention than normal hair, it certainly won't help you score points for terrific style in record time. So why not avoid that handicap by treating your hair kindly at the outset? Here your plastic-quill brush comes into play for the first time—starting not at the top of your head but at your nape. Part your hair off (horizontally) at the ears, and gently work the brush (or your wide-tooth comb if that's what you have) through the bottom layer; move upward as you gradually release more hair, always gently working out the tangles.

LOTIONS, POTIONS, AND OTHER BODYBUILDERS

It takes more than gentle handling, of course, to dry hair into eminently stylable form. Years ago hairdressers looked to lotions and lacquers to slick, stick, and glue hair into submission. They slathered their clients' hair with gobs of setting lotion, stuck them under dryers for an hour, and baked them crisp. Women had a tight curl that lasted three weeks, especially if they lacquered it enough. Well, that solved a problem back then. But today you want hair that looks and feels soft, swings loosely or tousles, moves with the wind (or with you) and then bounces back, holding its basic shape all day long. So the industry had to develop products that do essentially what the old ones did but within the context of today's feeling for hair.

Manufacturers have flooded the market with new formulas yielding hundreds of mousses, gels, lotions, and other fixatives to be sprayed, squeezed, smoothed, smeared, patted, pumped, and poured for every imaginable styling need. All are meant to help you control, direct, and maintain your hair without the wire-sculpture look and feel women used to get from setting lotions and lacquers.

I can't review the entire mind-boggling maze here. But a few guidelines should lead you to the right product group for a given purpose:

MOUSSES:

These are very light. They help you move the hair around easily and are great for giving soft styles direction. They also come to the aid of fine hair that cries out for extra body.

GELS:

Heavier than mousses, for general use, they're best in thicker, coarser, or curlier hair that needs more control and lifting power. I find a dab or two of Tenax excellent for controlling hair that tends to puff and frizz too much when it dries. Add just a tad more, and when it dries, you'll keep that shiny, wet look—great if you're into water sports or simply love the beach.

Even fine hair that needs extra strength at the temples or in some other area can benefit from a few strategically placed dabs of gel.

Apply mousses, gels, and other styling aids when your hair is still wet, directly from palms to areas that need the most attention.

HAIR SPRAYS:

Not to be confused with the old heavily lacquered "spray nets," they're no longer used to lock in or cement the hairstyle. Hair sprays still provide extra hold, but now they're light enough to use as a styling tool to help you get the look you want quickly.

GIVING YOUR HAIR A HEAD START

Just as mousses, gels, and sprays provide the muscle that gives your hair body, your blow-dryer gives it a warm-up. If you run, you warm up by stretching your muscles so your body will respond readily to the demands of a race. Why not give your hair the same edge? Successful hairstyles have volume *at the area closest to the root.* So even before you touch the ends, you want to direct or lift that root hair. And the warm-up to make your root hair respond readily begins with drying after a shampoo.

Most women struggle with a round styling brush and a blow-dryer, trying to curl the hair as they dry. But wet hair doesn't curl! It's silly to stand there for an hour stroking and rolling the same section over and over again, hitting it with heat repeatedly. It's worse than silly. It's a waste of your precious time. And even when you do get this terrific curl at the bottom, where's that volume you wanted? Volume comes directly from the root area (I can't repeat this often enough!), and you've spent all your time on the ends of your hair.

Instead, for sensational results fast, dry your hair immediately so you can get right to the styling step. The best way to do that is to bend forward, put your head down, and toss your hair over. Then blow it dry, using your fingers and your plastic-quill brush to separate the strands and keep the hair moving, while you keep the airflow moving with your other hand.

By letting your hair slide between your fingers now and then while it dries, you can feel any remaining tangles and gently work them out. And you can hold the root hair away from your scalp as you dry that section. This, incidentally, is your optimum chance to ensure maximum lift at your temples and correct stubborn cowlicks, parts, or waves. To accomplish any of these objectives, use your fingers to direct your hair where you want it to go.

With proper handling, your blow-dryer can be your greatest styling asset, starting with the many benefits that make upside-down drying the only sensible approach.

With your head down:

- your hair hangs loosely away from your scalp, inducing better airflow and, therefore, quicker drying than when it's clumped together and draped about your head.
- your blood circulates to your scalp, providing healthy stimulation you may not get standing upright.
- above all, your hair dries training the roots away from your scalp.

What results do you get? Toss your hair back, and see how much volume you have. You may think you look like fright night at the movies, but believe it or not, you've mastered the first step in gaining control over your hair.

Now use your fingers to place your hair essentially where you want it to go. If you've applied the right styling aids and blow-dried your hair properly, this step should be a breeze. Here again, *you* have control.

If it's necessary, use your blow-dryer with the plastic-quill brush to get added lift in specific areas. If you need some at the temples, for example, follow these steps:

1. With the brush in your right hand and the dryer in the other (or vice versa if you're left-handed), hold the brush with the quills facing your other arm.
2. Then slide only the first two rows of quills into the hair at your right temple (or left, depending on which hand holds the brush) in an upward direction, about an inch and a half.
3. Start applying heat from your dryer, and at the same time, slide the brush downward slightly (about a quarter of an inch) until you feel it catch the hair.
4. Then twist the brush, looping the hair around the first two rows (if you're twisting in the right direction, your thumb moves under and your knuckles rotate upward).
5. After you've twisted the brush, apply heat to that area for a few seconds, again keeping the nozzle moving.
6. Switch hands, and repeat the process for the other side.

What have you accomplished with this technique? You've guided the hair right from the roots in an upward direction. You've made it bend in a loop. And you've "set" the bend in with the dryer, producing a nice lift when you remove the brush.

This procedure works wherever lift and direction are needed—especially with short hair where you cover more territory. As you move toward the nape (for any length hair) rotate the quills upward. Then the steps are the same:

- Slide the brush into your hair.
- Bring it down slightly.
- Twist the brush in the direction you want your hair to go, wrapping the hair over those first two rows.
- Apply heat from your dryer for a few seconds.

For thicker, coarser, or curlier hair you might have more success with this procedure using the vented brush. Or *you may find it easier to use your fingers instead of a brush.* And you can get a similar result. A big advantage here: You have only one tool to handle, eliminating the need to manipulate brush and dryer simultaneously:

- Just slide your fingers into your hair.
- Curl them and grip the hair.
- Twist your hand as you would the brush with your knuckles going back toward the scalp and your fingertips rotating outward.
- Apply hot air.

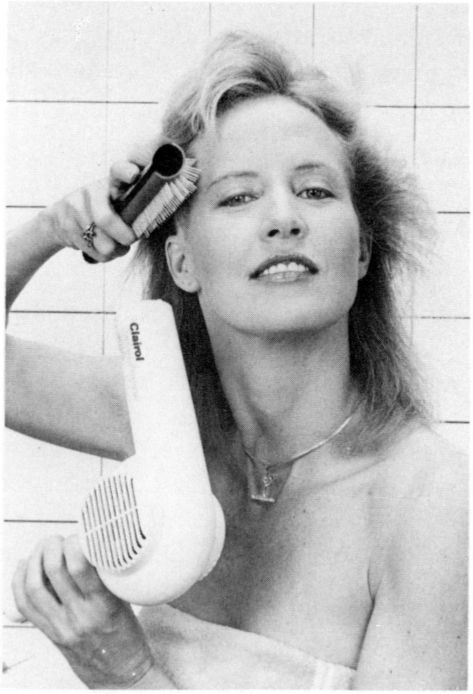

1

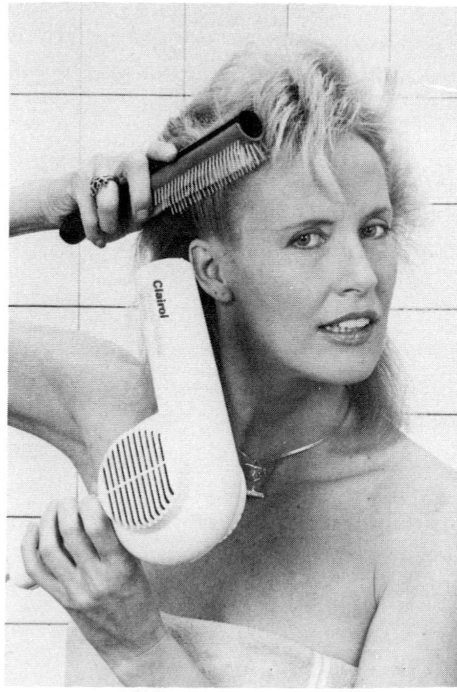

2

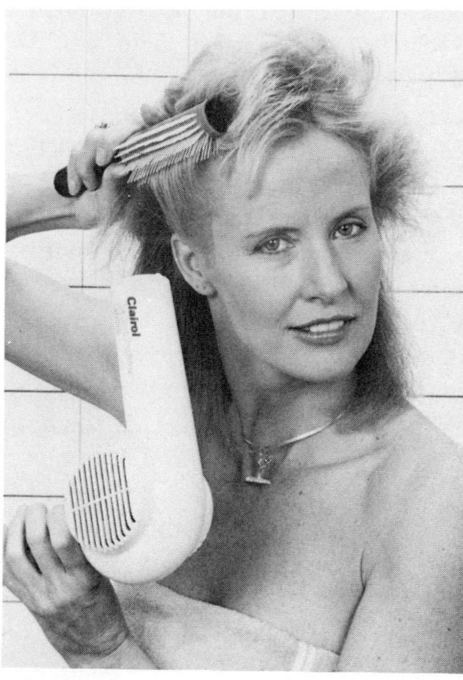

3

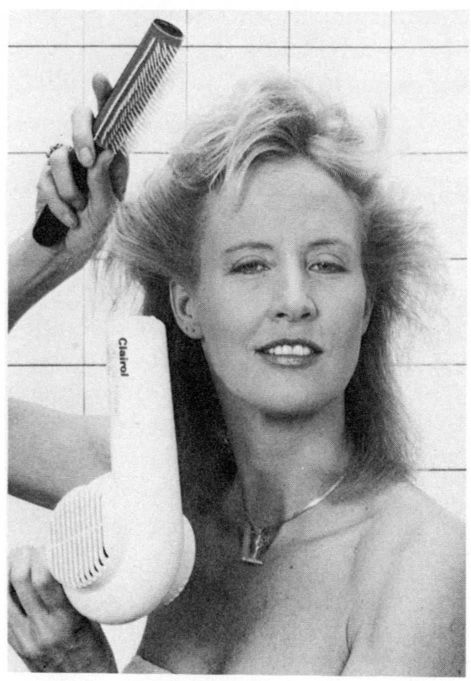

4

Whichever tool you prefer, with just a bit of practice (your temples are the best training ground), you'll soon run all the steps into one continuous motion that takes mere seconds to complete. And in mastering this maneuver, you will have mastered the basis for any hairstyle: lift, bend, direction, and control.

Team a blow-dryer with a round brush, and you have yet another styling technique. You can use it, as you would a roller, to create a soft curl or a wave here and there (only in dry hair, remember). The size of the bend you'll get depends on the size of your brush. But if you need a full set, it makes no sense to set your entire head, section by section, with a round brush and blow-dryer when you can get the same result or better ten times faster with hot rollers.

Surprisingly, even many professionals haven't learned this, for some reason. It never ceases to amaze me to see a colleague stand behind a client (who already has two or three round brushes sticking out of her head), waving a blow-dryer around while he struggles to balance yet a few more brushes under his arms and between his knees.

The brush does have practical applications. If you want curve at your nape or curl at your cheeks, your round brush can create it. In fact, you can use it to get soft touches at the ends of your hair almost anywhere you need them.

Another useful function for this tool is to relax a curl that's too tight, to stretch it, reshape it into a larger curl pattern. Just roll the brush into your hair, and apply heat from your dryer while you gradually exert gentle pressure on the brush to slide it out of the curl.

MAKING WAVES

If you really want to make waves or curls, *instant hot rollers* are far better than the blow-dryer and brush. Women often ask me, "Can I put them in wet hair?" or "Shouldn't I use mist rollers?" My answer to both questions: Why would you want to? I mean, what's the point of drying your hair only to wet it again? Setting hair from wet to dry for a firmer, tighter curl, if you recall, is an outdated approach, and it probably won't give you the result you want in view of today's hairstyles. Besides, these are the things that slow you up, and our whole purpose is to help you learn how to style your hair fashionably but quickly.

Since you already have that lift and bounce because of the way you dried your hair earlier, all you need are a few strategically placed rollers to enhance your hairstyle.

Actually, if you have a routine, using heated rollers can be your quickest way out of the house in the morning. Just heat the unit while you shower, for example, bend your head forward, and dry your hair fast. Throw a few rollers in where needed: two or three on top for short hair; a few at the bottom for long hair. Apply your makeup, brush out your set, and—*voilà*—you're done!

If you're an out-of-bed out-of-the-house person, tired of the same old wash-and-wear hairstyle, spot touch-ups with a *curling iron,* which can heat while you're dressing, could help you vary short hair. Don't even think of using this appliance to set your entire head if you want to get away from your mirror in five minutes.

The wand consists of two parts: the curling barrel and the spring-release clip, a curved arm that hugs the barrel. Whichever way you want to wind your curl, face the clip in the opposite direction or you'll create a ridge in your curl pattern. For example, if you want your curl to wind back, face the clip forward; if you want your curl to wind under, face the clip upward. Hold the section of hair away from your scalp, and with the clip pressed open, slide the wand onto your hair. Release the clip, and when the wand has grabbed your hair, slide it gently to the end, and roll. Hold for anywhere from five to fifteen seconds, depending how hot your iron gets. Press the spring release, and gently remove the wand.

Yet another convenient curling appliance is the *electric styling brush.* It looks like the curling iron, but its soft, flexible teeth, which grip the hair, make rolling easier for some. Clairol's latest model has a release button that also makes unrolling a breeze after you've set in the curl. This appliance, too, should be used for spot touch-ups. Place the wand partway up the section of hair; brush it to the end; then roll it up. Hold for a few seconds to let the heat do its job. Press the release button, and gently roll it out.

STYLING TIPS

These hints will upgrade your results from merely superb to sensational!

Backbrushing and backcombing can give you firmer hold and more control. But don't confuse either technique with old-fashioned teasing, which involved really packing the hair down to the roots.

When I was learning to style hair, most women looked as if their heads were too big for their bodies—thanks to the three Bs: beehives, bouffants, and bubbles. To achieve that look, we had to learn how to tease hair, and the acid test for a sufficiently packed-in tease was performed with knitting needles. You stuck them into the bulbous mound of hair in front of you, gave a tug, and if they didn't budge, you had it.

Today, thank heaven, we need no knitting needles to test the merits of styling techniques. Gentle backbrushing would never pass the knitting-needle test, but it sure comes in handy to perk up a style or blend a set. What if your hair, which had been set in rollers earlier, separated into the individual set formation during the day? You blend those curls with *backbrushing:*

1. Hold the hair away from the scalp.
2. Using your small paddle brush, lightly stroke the surface layer, starting from about an inch and a half from the scalp, and push forward in short, sweeping motions.

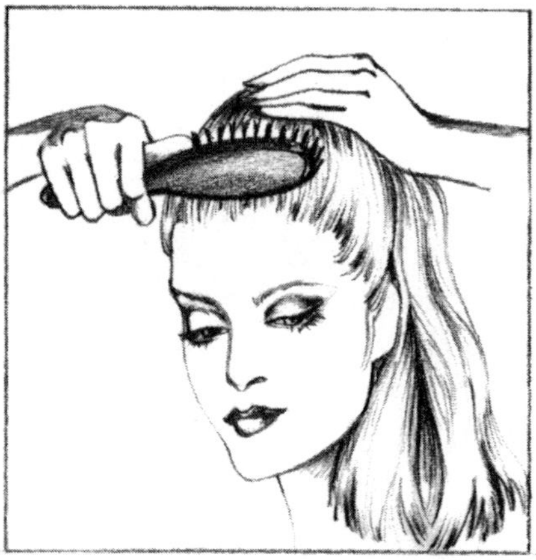

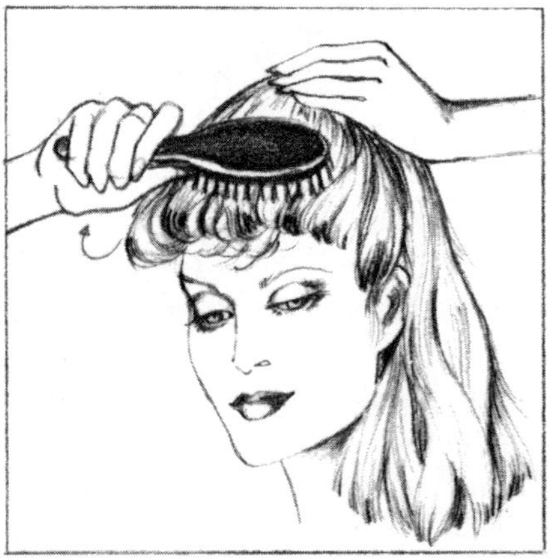

3. Slide back to the next section, and repeat the process.
4. Then use the edges of the brush or your fingertips to blend ends into place.

Your hair still should be soft and natural enough to put your fingers through it so you can place and arrange it easily.

- *Backcombing* works well when a hairstyle needs extra support. Say, the great upward sweep you had at the temples has fizzled.

1. Holding your hair up, work your comb lightly in short, circular strokes, again on the surface layer.

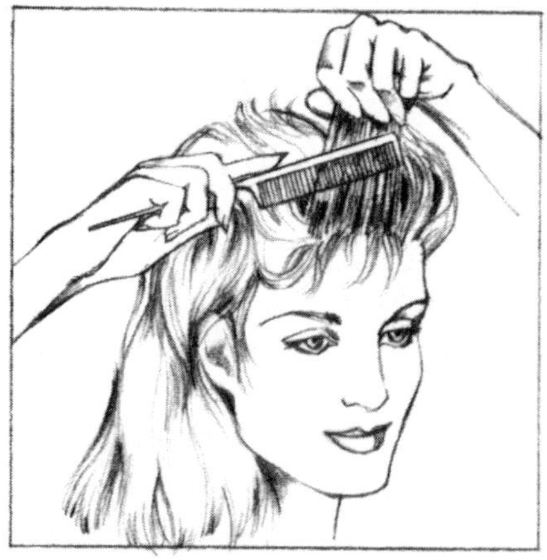

   Start about an inch from the scalp, and push forward.
2. Use the pick (or tail) end of your comb to smooth hair into place.

- You can *achieve several effects with a vented brush:* Take short, layered hair that runs from straight to wavy as an example. Rake your vented brush through it for added surface texture. Or you can enhance the line of a wedged or stacked haircut simply by blowing it dry forward as usual and then brushing it back with the vented brush.
- *Hair spray,* as I mentioned earlier, not only provides extra hold when you're done but makes a great styling aid applied after your hair is dried or during the course of the day. For example, is your layered hair dropping at the crown? Slide your fingers into your hair, and gently lift from the roots.

Spray with a nonaerosol extra- or firm-hold hair spray, and scrunch your hair with your fingers. The result is more lift and texture, but you've achieved both in seconds instead of spending ten minutes to place your hair, then spraying it.

I like Final Net, one of many nonsticky hair sprays available today for quick hands-on techniques like this one.

SOME THOUGHTS ABOUT DEXTERITY

By now you should have a pretty clear idea of which tools, appliances, and styling aids will help you make your hair behave as you want it to. And you should have some insight into how to make them produce those results fast. But I can't tell you which ones you'll use most comfortably. Dexterity, like every human capability, is highly individual, and our ease or difficulty in handling implements varies. That's why manufacturers have developed so many different tools and appliances that essentially do the same job.

Ideally you should try using a tool once or twice before buying it. But that's not always realistic. You can't "test-drive" appliances to see how they handle. However, you can ask your hairdresser to let you try a few of his or hers. Or perhaps your friends own items similar to those you're considering and wouldn't mind your giving them a whirl.

While you don't need incredible coordination to use any of the tools I described, you may have to practice just a bit to become totally proficient with them. And why not? You wouldn't expect to swoosh down even a beginner's slope your first few times on skis.

So, if you have to invest extra time up front to develop your hair-managing skills, don't despair. Just think of the long-term gain your investment will yield—and go for it!

LENGTH & TEXTURE	WAVE PATTERN	DETANGLE WET HAIR	DRY DAMP HAIR	SHAPE & STYLE ALMOST DRY HAIR	FINISH DRY HAIR
SHORT—COARSE	WAVY TO CURLY	VENTED	VENTED	ROUND	VENTED
	WAVY TO STRAIGHT	VENTED	VENTED	ROUND	VENTED
SHORT—MEDIUM	WAVY TO CURLY	VENTED	VENTED	ROUND	VENTED
	WAVY TO STRAIGHT	PLASTIC QUILL	PLASTIC QUILL	PLASTIC QUILL	VENTED
SHORT—FINE	WAVY TO CURLY	PLASTIC QUILL	PLASTIC QUILL	PLASTIC QUILL	VENTED
	WAVY TO STRAIGHT	PLASTIC QUILL	PLASTIC QUILL	PLASTIC QUILL	VENTED
MEDIUM—COARSE	WAVY TO CURLY	PLASTIC QUILL	VENTED	PLASTIC QUILL	VENTED
	WAVY TO STRAIGHT	PLASTIC QUILL	PLASTIC QUILL	PLASTIC QUILL	VENTED
MEDIUM—MEDIUM	WAVY TO CURLY	PLASTIC QUILL	PLASTIC QUILL	VENTED	VENTED
	WAVY TO STRAIGHT	PLASTIC QUILL	PLASTIC QUILL	PLASTIC QUILL	VENTED
MEDIUM—FINE	WAVY TO CURLY	PLASTIC QUILL	PLASTIC QUILL	ROUND	FINGERS*
	WAVY TO STRAIGHT	PLASTIC QUILL	PLASTIC QUILL	ROUND	FINGERS*
LONG—COARSE	WAVY TO CURLY	PLASTIC QUILL	FINGERS*1	PLASTIC QUILL	FINGERS
	WAVY TO STRAIGHT	PLASTIC QUILL	PLASTIC QUILL	ROUND*2	FINGERS
LONG—MEDIUM	WAVY TO CURLY	PLASTIC QUILL	FINGERS	PLASTIC QUILL	FINGERS
	WAVY TO STRAIGHT	PLASTIC QUILL	PLASTIC QUILL	ROUND	PADDLE BRUSH
LONG—FINE	WAVY TO CURLY	PLASTIC QUILL	FINGERS*3	PLASTIC QUILL	FINGERS
	WAVY TO STRAIGHT	PLASTIC QUILL	PLASTIC QUILL	ROUND	PADDLE BRUSH

NOTE: IN SHORTER HAIRSTYLES WHERE WE WANT TO ENHANCE TEXTURE FOR MORE EXCITING LOOKS, THE VENTED BRUSH CAN BE USED TO FINISH DRY HAIR TO GIVE A VARIEGATED FEELING FOR THE LAYERS—LIKE SLIDING FINGERS THROUGH THE HAIR.

NOTE: WHEN SHAPING & STYLING ALMOST DRY HAIR, IT IS COMMON TO LAY THE BRUSH DOWN TEMPORARILY TO USE FINGERS.
* FINE HAIR SHOULD ALWAYS BE TREATED AS GENTLY AS SILK. FINISH DRY HAIR WITH FINGERS TO ENHANCE VOLUME WHERE ANY TYPE OF BRUSH WOULD DECREASE THE VOLUME.

*1 UNLESS WANTING TO STRETCH CURL, USE PLASTIC QUILL.
*2 IF MORE CURL & BEND ARE DESIRED.
*3 I PREFER TO USE FINGERS ON HAIR THAT TENDS TO HAVE A WAVE OR A CURL. THIS METHOD WILL EXPAND THE CURL—WHERE A BRUSH WOULD LOOSEN IT.

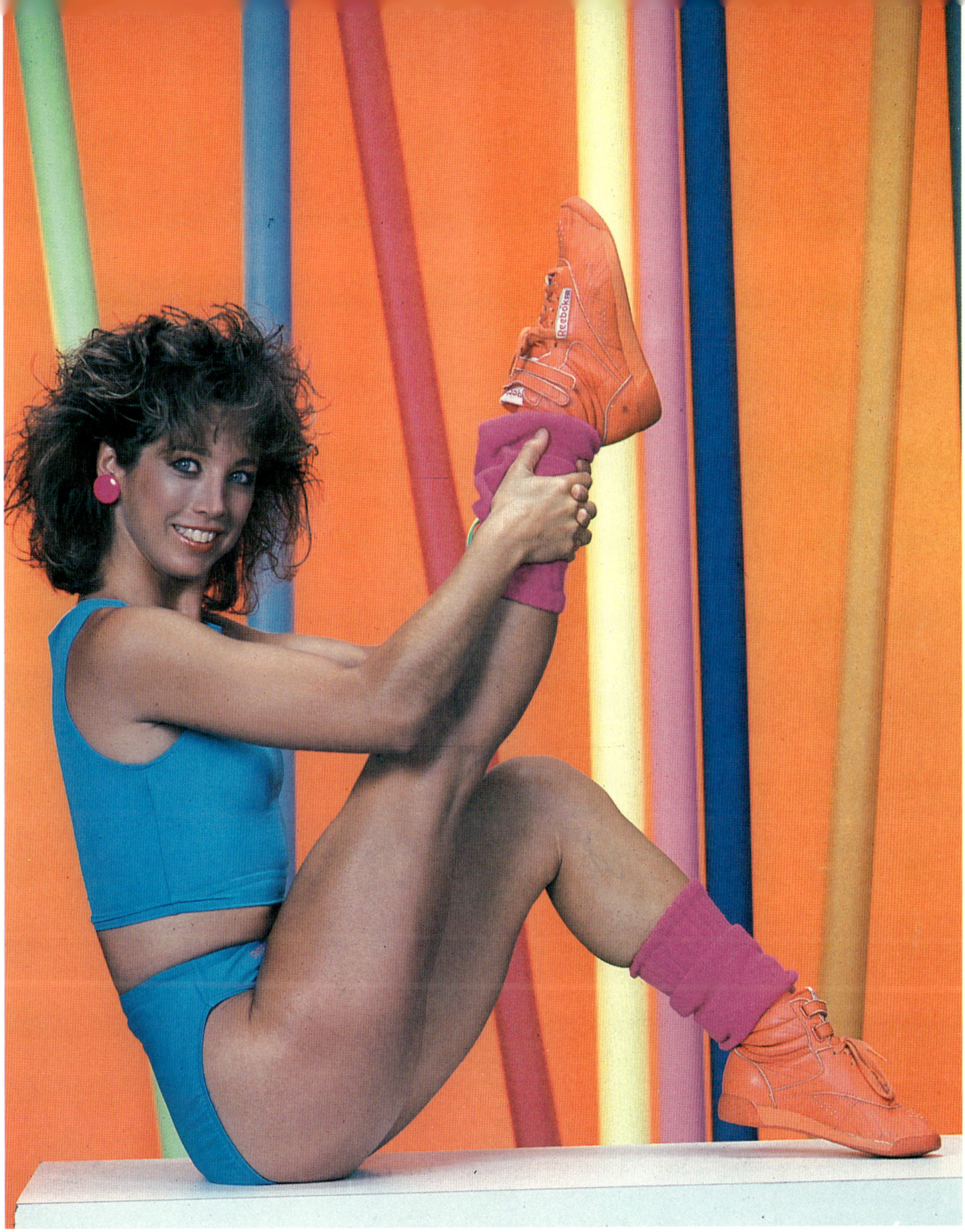

DENISE AUSTIN

Aerobics whiz Denise Austin, a regular on NBC-TV's "Today" show who also heads her own consulting firm which places fitness programs with corporations, finds that her medium-textured, wavy hair, kept all one length with layering around her face, gives her the glamorous hairstyles she wants with minimum fuss.

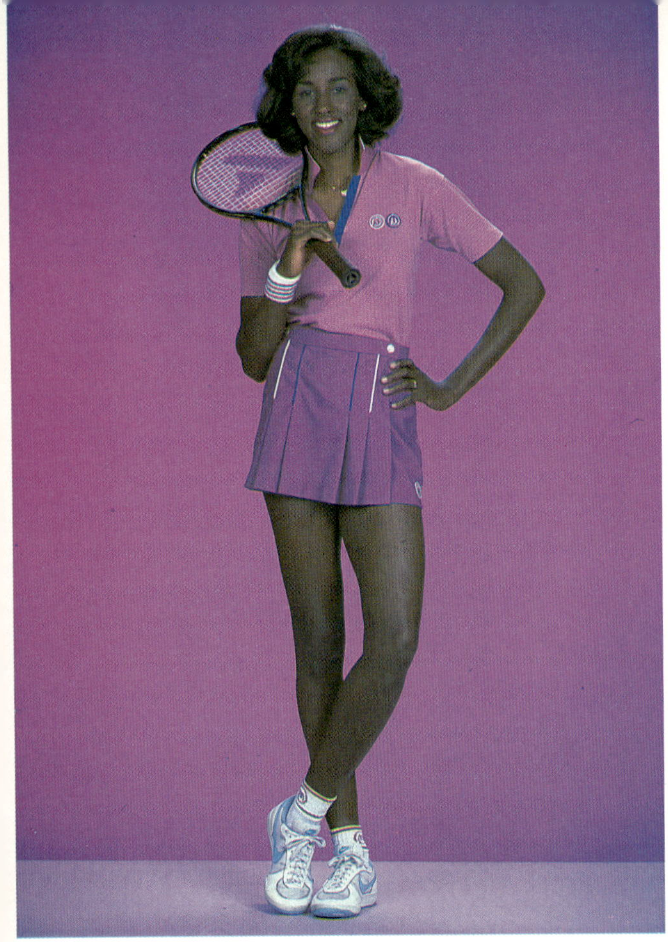

LESLIE ALLEN

Leslie Allen, who in 1981 became the first black woman to win a major tennis tournament (the $125,000 Avon purse) since Althea Gibson's 1958 Wimbledon and U.S. Open victories, credits modern hair-relaxing techniques for the hairstyling versatility she enjoys despite her busy, strenuous schedule.

APRIL ALLEN

Having won ten national and four world roller-skating championships, April Allen has put her talents to work on the Broadway stage in hits such as *The Rink, Singin' in the Rain,* and *Starlight Express.* Permanent waving for body allows her the flexibility to create the many different looks her career and private life demand.

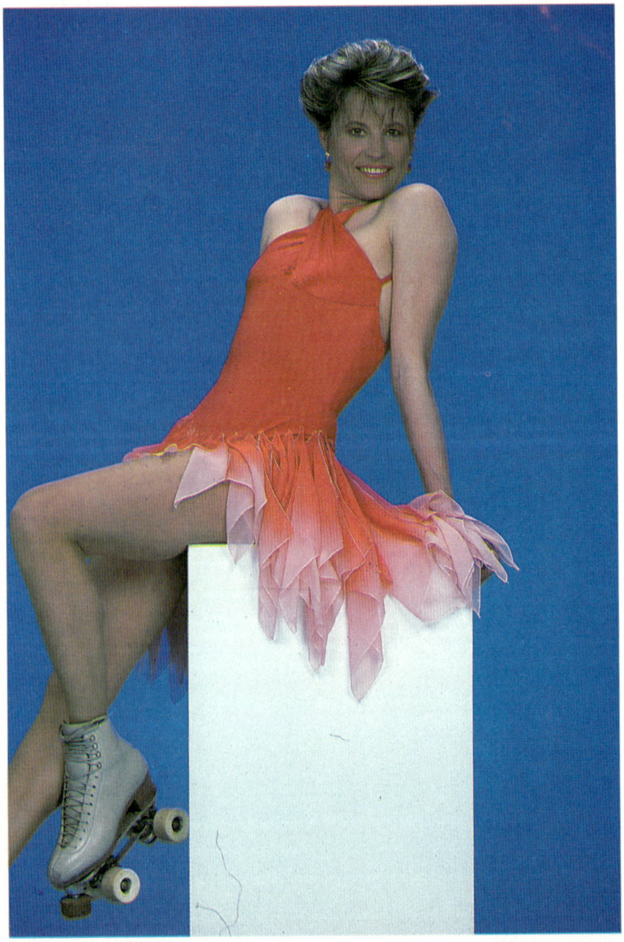

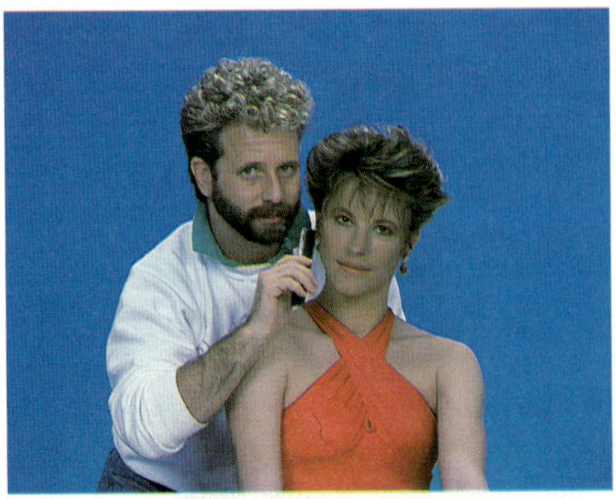

JUDY BLUMBERG

Judy Blumberg, who with her skating partner Michael Seibert has won the U.S. Ice Dance Championship five times, uses highlighting to enhance the color and texture of her short, layered hair.

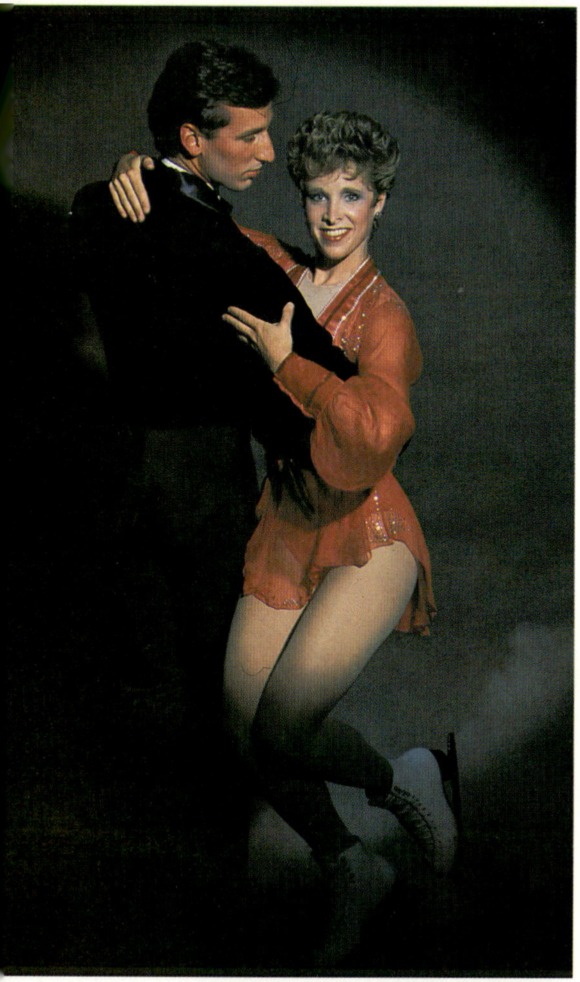

SUZY CHAFFEE

Three-time world freestyle skiing champion and Olympic team captain turned film star Suzy Chaffee also devotes her energies to active support of women's sports and business interests, including resort development and her own line of women's skis. She feels that permanent waving has helped make hairstyling much easier for her multi-faceted way of life.

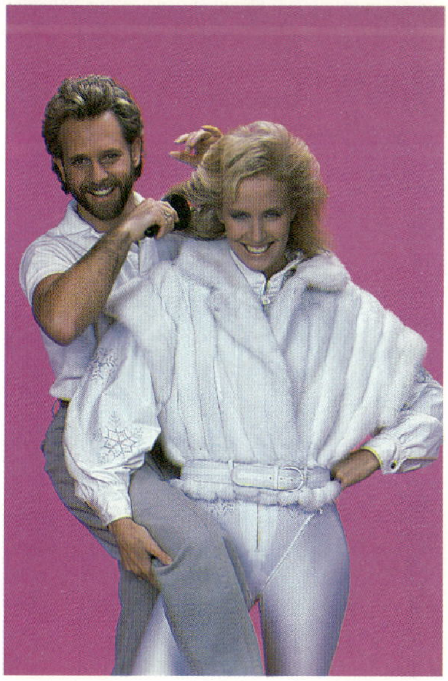

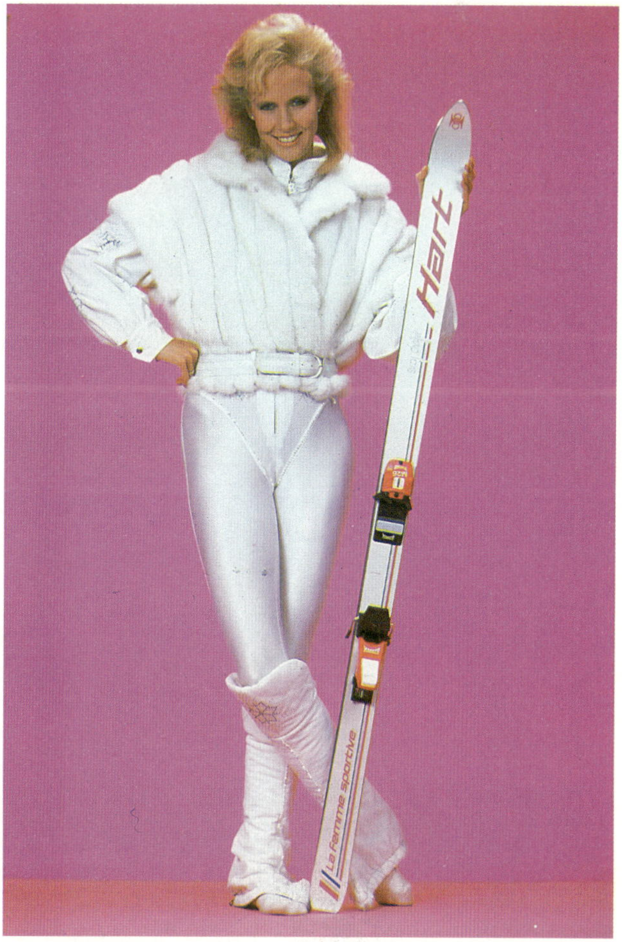

JENNIFER CHANDLER

Jennifer Chandler, who in 1976 won the Olympic Gold Medal for her graceful, balletlike diving, has medium-textured, wavy hair which many consider ideal—especially for active women—because it tends to offer the greatest number of styling options and needs the least amount of coaxing to achieve most of them.

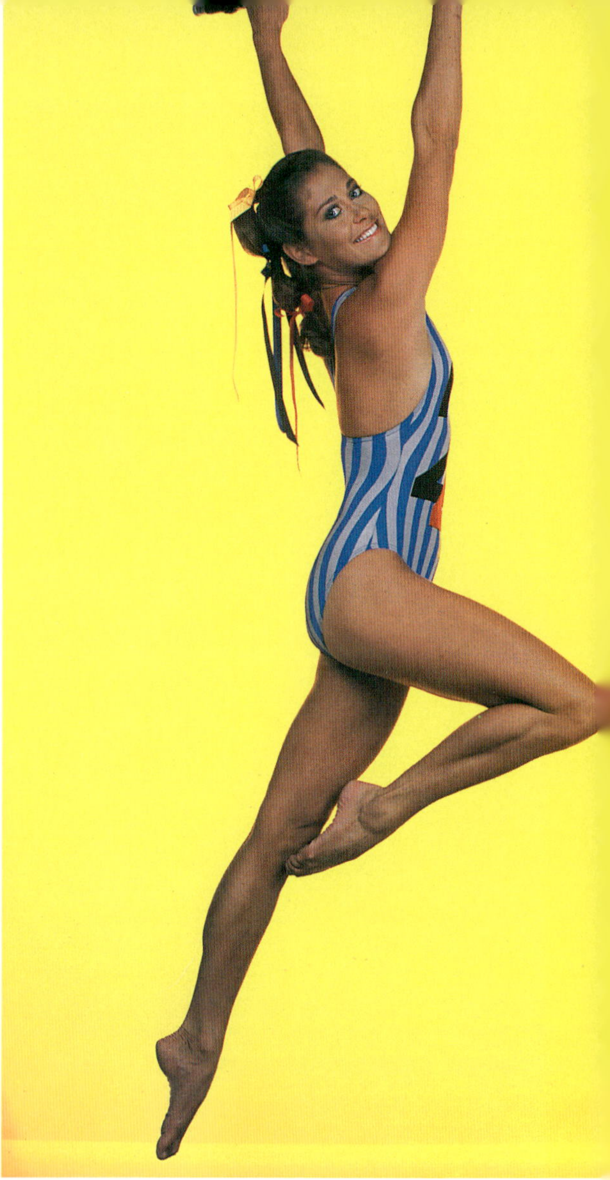

CANDY COSTIE

In 1984 Candy Costie and her synchronized swimming partner Tracie Ruiz snapped up the coveted Olympic Gold for its first-ever synchronized swimming duet event. Candy manages to keep her constantly immersed hair at high-performance level with scrupulous attention to conditioning.

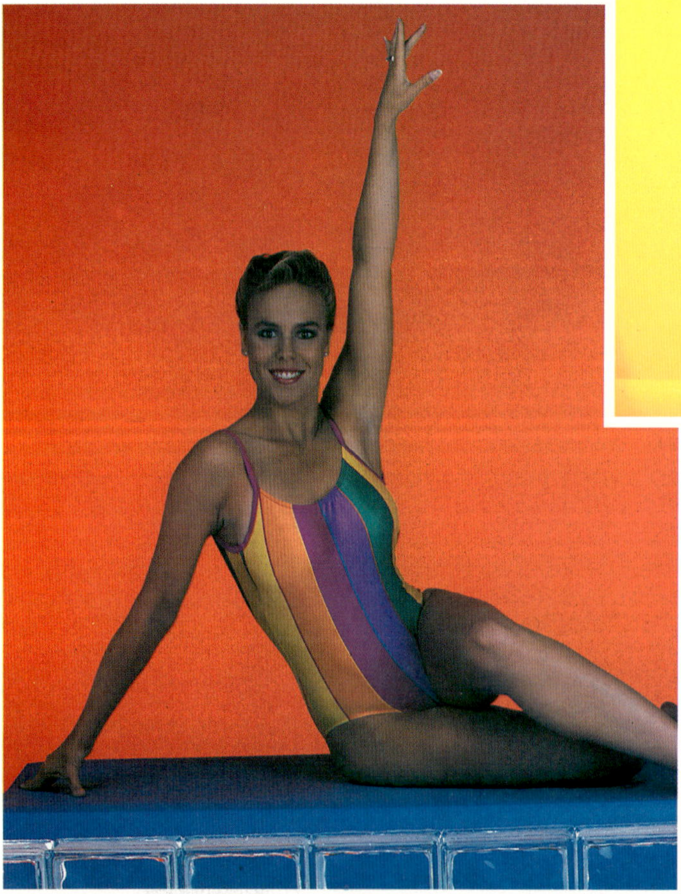

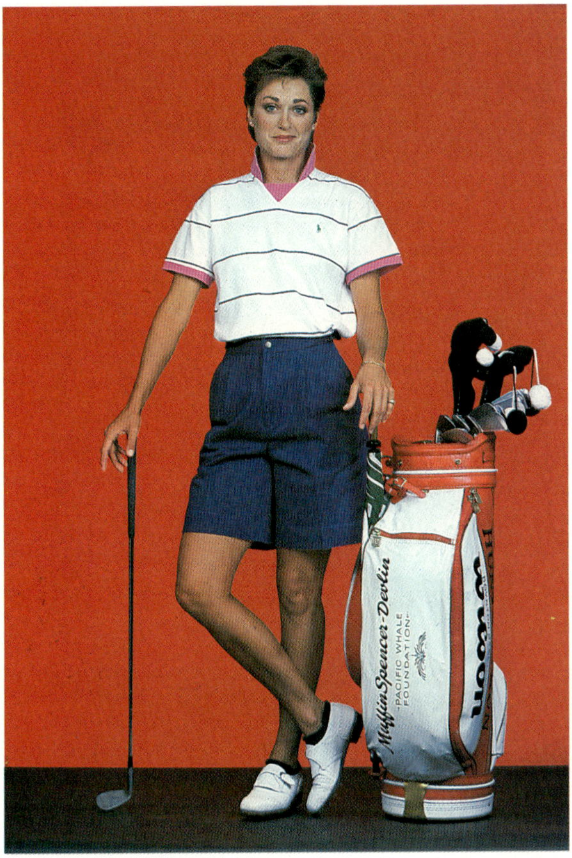

MUFFIN SPENCER-DEVLIN

A late bloomer in women's professional golf, Muffin Spencer-Devlin has enjoyed a striking success since she joined the LPGA tour in 1979. Although her hair is ultra-short, she can vary her look to suit the demands of her life on and off the golf course.

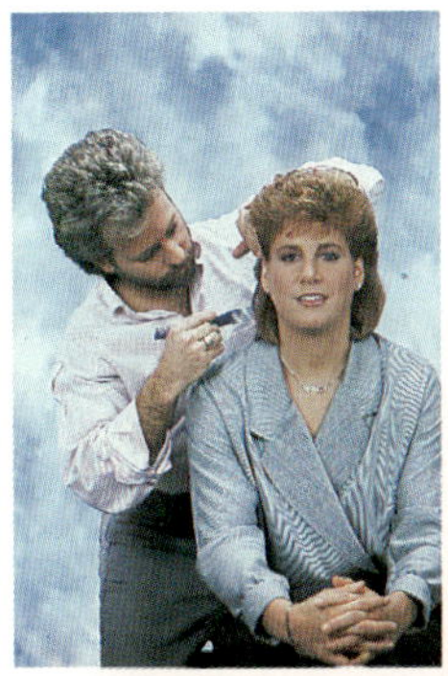

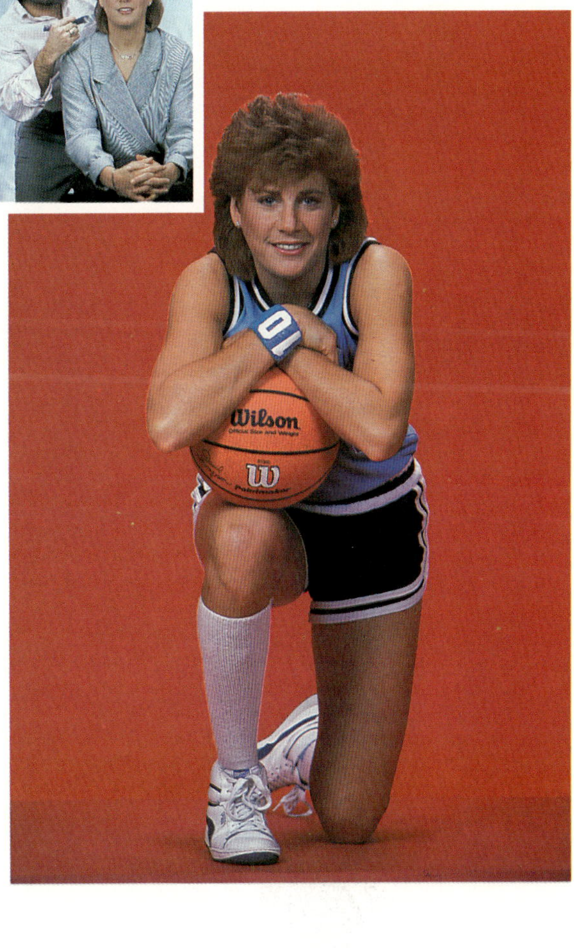

NANCY LIEBERMAN

A Silver Medalist for women's basketball in the 1976 Olympics and winner of the Gold Medal at the Pan American Games in 1975, Nancy Lieberman now plays championship basketball for the Dallas Diamonds. She feels that having high performance hair—maintained, in her case, with the help of a body wave—can add the extra edge of confidence it takes to make a winner.

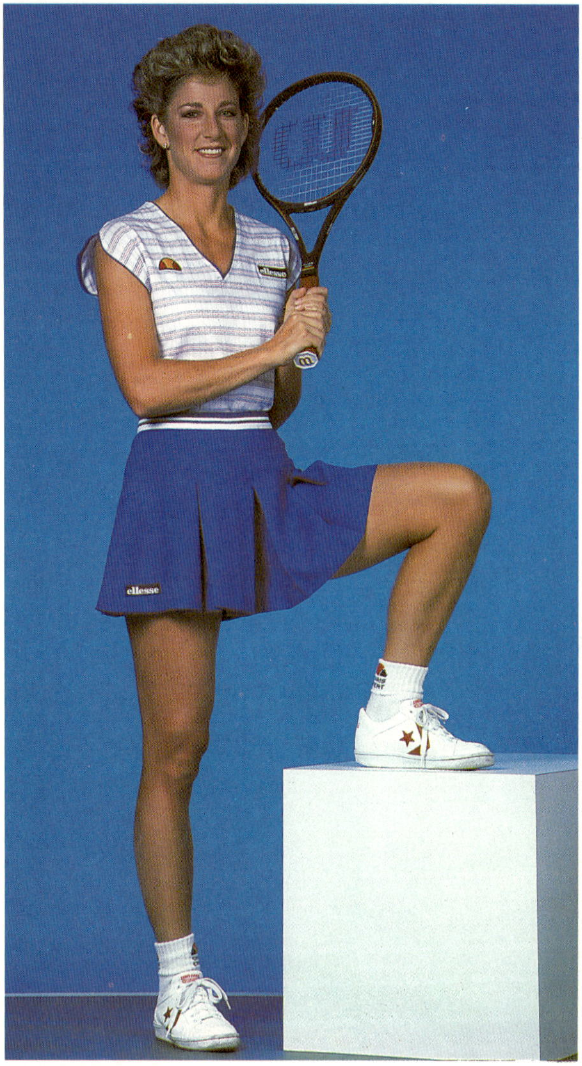

CHRIS EVERT LLOYD

Chris Evert Lloyd, six-time U.S. Open winner, who broke an important barrier in women's tennis when she became the first female player to reach the million-dollar mark in tournament earnings, depends on permanent waving and highlighting to help keep her fine hair at high-performance level.

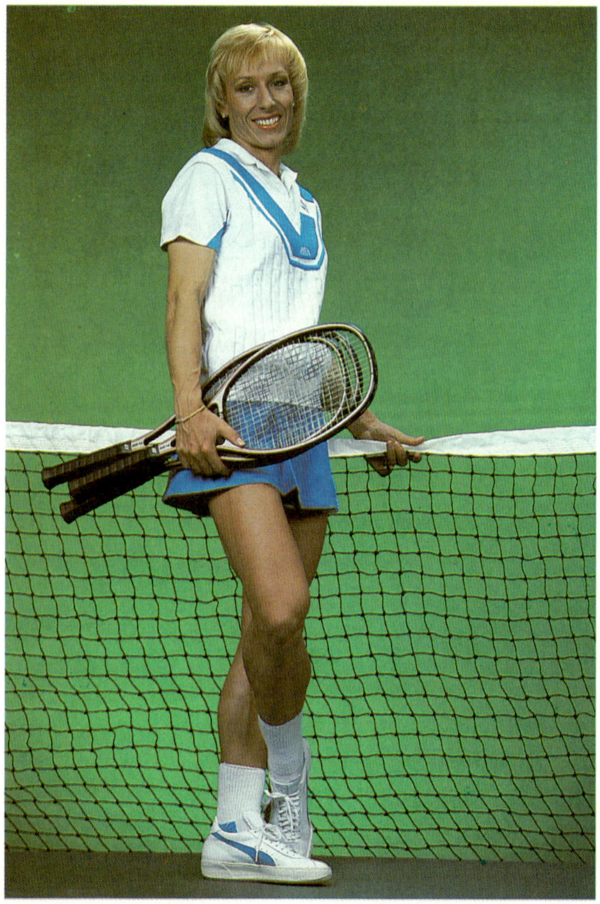

MARTINA NAVRATILOVA

Martina Navratilova, who, with total tournament earnings by 1986 reported at over $10 million, has won more prize money than any other tennis professional—male or female, traded her once-famous ponytail for striking blond hair cut to move with her on the tennis court and to give her considerable hairstyling flexibility.

DEBI THOMAS

1986 Women's World Figure Skating Champion Debi Thomas—the first black ice skater to snag the top honor in a world singles competition—also strives for high performance in Stanford University's premed program. Her short, layered hair—with some length at the back—provides the comfort, versatility and handling ease to satisfy the hairstyling demands of her varied and grueling schedule.

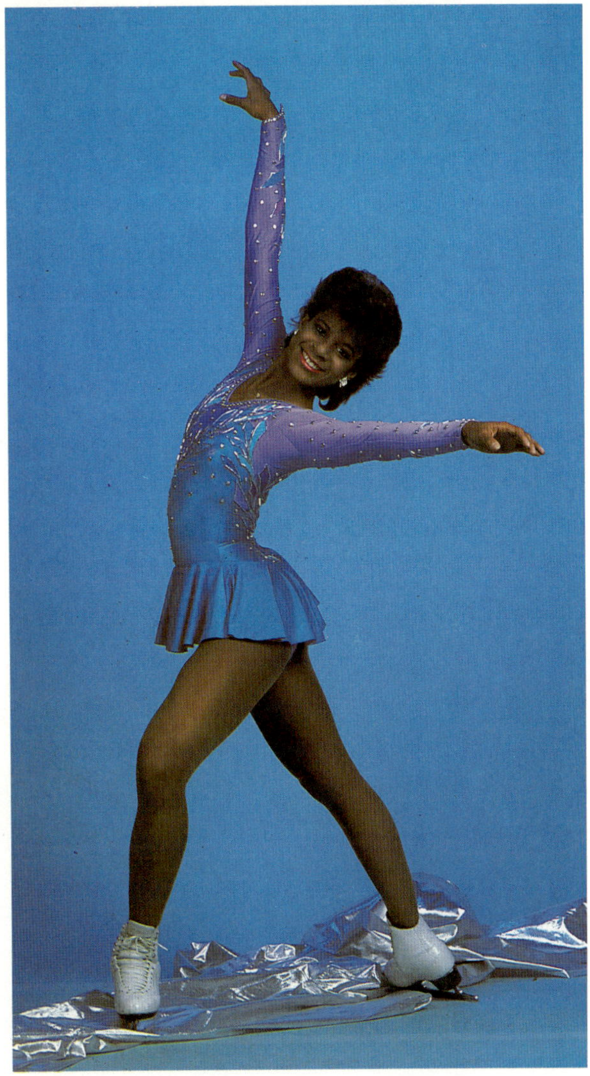

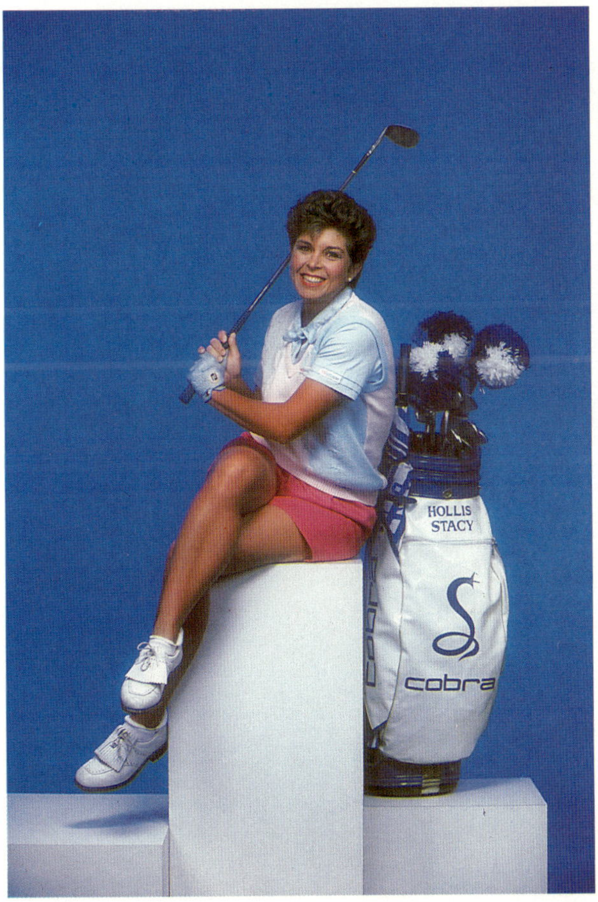

HOLLIS STACY

Three-time U.S. Open winner in women's golf Hollis Stacy, noted for repeating her victories (as she also did with the West Virginia Classic, the S&H Golf Classic, and the CPC International) is said to be one of the LPGA's most flamboyant performers. She makes use of stubborn cowlicks rather than trying to fight them to achieve her high performance hairstyles.

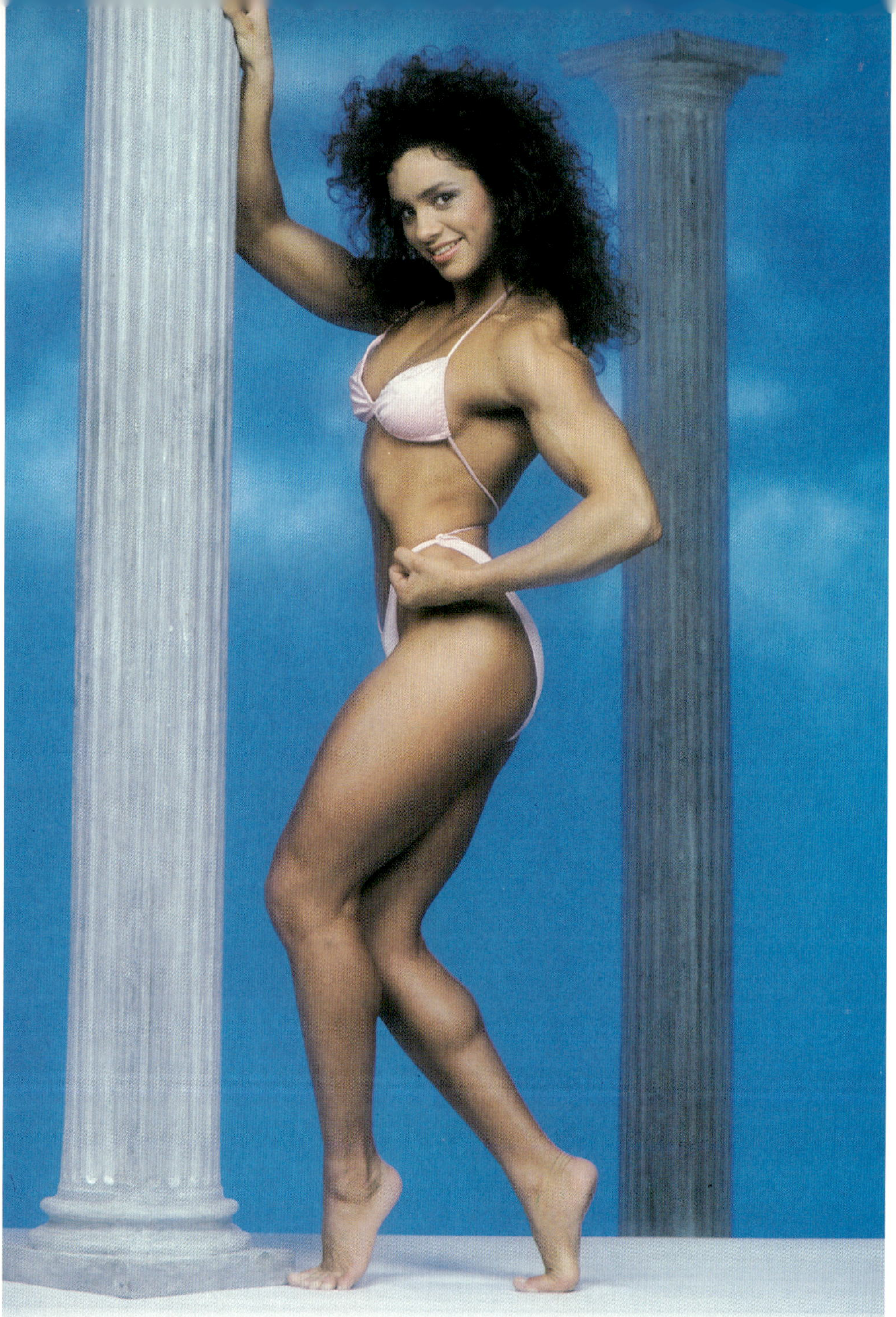

GLADYS PORTUGUES

Gladys Portugues, who was featured in the film *Pumping Iron II: The Women* and has appeared on the covers of national magazines ranging from *Sports Style* and *Flex* to *Ms., Self,* and *Cosmopolitan's Beauty Guide,* layers her thick, coarse hair in order to keep it long and at high-performance level.

SIX

SHORT CUTS: NOT YOUR ONLY SHORTCUT TO HIGH PERFORMANCE HAIR

I have never believed that an active or athletic life-style demands short-cropped hair. Yet so many active women keep their hair short strictly because they're convinced it's the only easy hair care option for a hectic schedule.

I realize that a hectic schedule doesn't necessarily include sports. But I cite female athletes to illustrate my point because they rank among the most active women I know. And quite a few are opting for longer hair these days. If *they* can make it work within the context of their strenuous pace, surely so can you!

True, full-time sportswomen once found a practical solution in boyish haircuts because short hair *is* easy and doesn't get in the way during competition. But neither does it earn Brownie points for femininity, versatility, or graceful, flattering movement. And with ever-expanding television coverage of women's sports catapulting female athletes into the world spotlight, many now want hair that has all those characteristics, largely for that extra touch of glamour virtually anytime they might be seen.

That is not to say you can't look wonderful and feminine in short hair. Golf pro Muffin Spencer-Devlin's appearance clearly refutes any such notion (see photos pages 125–127). Her structured cut has marvelous contrasting texture in light, airy wisps that flow through a graceful wave on top into sleek sides and back. The combination focuses lots of attention on her lovely features, especially complimenting her expressive eyes and mouth and highlighting her graceful neck. If you, like Muffin, look and feel fabulous in short hair, by all means wear yours short! But if that isn't your best look, don't consider it your only alternative, practical though it may be.

You only have to glance at the sports personalities featured in this book to know that even for athletes, "practical" no longer describes a haircut that merely keeps hair out of the way. Certainly this feature counts in competition. But to be truly practical, a haircut also must flatter a sports star during the height of frenetic movement when all eyes gaze in her direction. Equally important, it must allow her to vary her look to suit her life outside the sporting arena. And it must need little, if any, coaxing to do all this in what scant time she has between trains and planes, competition and other work-related commitments, and the demands of her private life, which aren't unlike those you face.

Your own life, uncelebrated though it may be in the strictest sense, probably seems just as frenetic at times as any athlete's, and that's precisely the point. Of course, you don't play as much tennis, golf, or whatever as sports celebrities do. Maybe you don't indulge in sports at all. But if you take yoga lessons, attend aerobic dance classes, work out to your favorite exercise video, or simply find yourself constantly running from car pools, to a job, to school board meetings and who knows what other chores and interests that fill your life, you, too, need a high performance cut that makes you feel admired by the public *you* deal with every day.

A high performance haircut has several properties:

- *It enhances what nature gave you, using your hair's natural inclination to its best advantage.* If your hair is wavy or curly, a high performance cut will make the most of your waves or curls. If it's straight, it will turn your hair into a wonderful sculptured silhouette. In either case, with a high performance cut your hair will assume a marvelous shape—*even when it's wet.*

  In my opinion, that's the true test of a haircut. When a client's hair is freshly cut and still wet, I know immediately that it's going to work. In fact, often that's precisely when clients ask, "Why can't my hair always have this look?"

  If you swim or indulge in water sports, you should feel good about your hair when it's wet. Then invest five minutes of styling time with a blow-dryer, and it can only get better. Five minutes more, and it should look better yet. In other words, with a high performance cut, your hairstyle will improve with attention, but your hair shouldn't need much attention to look pretty terrific in the first place.

- *A high performance cut makes styling almost effortless.* Hollis Stacy's medium-fine, straight hair has lots of cowlicks. But when her hair is wet, she can mold it into almost any shape she likes, with a little help from a gel or a mousse, which gives her extra control over her hair. Like Hollis, even if you have straight hair, with a high performance cut you should be able to move it around and guide it into a flattering shape using the right styling aids and very little effort on your part.

- *A high performance cut gives you the flexibility to change your hairstyle when the mood or need arises.* Even short hair should provide the option to wear it brought forward, for example, for a softer look or slicked back for a sleeker line, with a third option, perhaps, in some combination of the two.
- *A high performance cut gives you hairstyles that need little, if any, maintenance through the day or evening.* Actually you shouldn't even have to think about your hair much, let alone fuss with it—whether it's kinky, straight, or somewhere in between. After all, why wouldn't hair that "shapes up" when it's wet do at least as well as, if not better than, that for you as it gradually moves back toward its natural state during the course of your activities?
- *A high performance cut lets your hair move with you, doesn't get in your way, and falls back into a semblance of its original shape afterward.* Skating star Dorothy Hamill's famous haircut demonstrates this quality better than any I can think of. During those high-speed spins that hair whips right around with her without disrupting her balance one iota. Then, when she whirls to a stop, it swings gracefully into place.

How can you help your hairdresser design a high performance cut for you? By communicating your needs and desires to him or her clearly. That means you must carefully evaluate those needs first.

When Martina Navratilova decided to acquire a new look, I knew she had given the matter a great deal of thought beforehand. She didn't know how her hair should be cut, of course, but she knew precisely what she wanted it to do. And that made it a lot easier for me to get a result gratifying to both of us. I have to assume that since at this writing she hasn't changed her style in more than three years, the cut has served her well.

Before the change her hair had appeared constrained because it was clipped back and caught in elastic bands, especially when she was most visible—on the tennis court. The look clearly contradicted Martina's personality as an aggressive player whose strong, fast-paced maneuvers exude lots of power. But if she hadn't worn that ponytail, her below-shoulder-length hair would have obstructed her during competition.

What's more, in Martina's case, all-one-length hair didn't offer much in the way of versatility, and pulled back, it did nothing to enhance her angular features.

She wanted her hair as long as possible yet in a style that didn't need four barrettes and elastic bands to keep it out of her way. To achieve this, I cut her hair to the collarline, layering it so it could hang loosely without a length of hair anywhere that could get in her eyes no matter how she moved. With all one length, even at the collarline, the strands on top would have whipped across her face while she played.

Finally, I gave her some soft wisps around the edges, which, with her hair brought forward to frame her face, flatter Martina's almost sculptured features.

Does her haircut fulfill her need for a versatile, easy-wear, easy-care hairstyle?

"It's totally comfortable and takes me five minutes to do," Martina told a Long Island *Newsday* reporter, adding that with the help of a few hot rollers she easily can turn that basic style into a dressier evening look (see photos page 73).

Does it move with her on the tennis court? Does it enhance her movements? You have only to see her in action to decide for yourself.

The real issue here is that you, too, must walk into that salon with a fair idea of what you'd like your hair to do for you—functionally as well as aesthetically—if you want your hairstylist's peak performance with those scissors.

Okay, so maybe you don't rank among the neighborhood superjocks. That simply gives you a wider range of choices than someone like Martina has. After all, even if you do play tennis often, bowl once a week, or run every morning, a ponytail could suit you to a tee for the hour or so you give to that kind of recreational activity. And there're always headbands. Not only are they functional for many athletes, but headbands can be chic, too. Remember Olivia Newton-John in her video (with its decidedly athletic theme) "Let's Get Physical!"

Actually many an active woman finds long hair the easiest to manage if she pops a headband around it or catches it all back in a covered elastic band, then undoes it later, throws in a few hot rollers for five minutes, and brushes it out.

What works for you is what counts in this decision, but you must have a fair idea of what that is. Do you garden, help out with tots in a local day care center, bike ride, picnic with your family, take your kids to a playground every day, or travel a lot on business? If you do any of these activities, they should play a part in your choice of a haircut.

Another issue to consider: Where do you work? Today most companies allow employees to set their own grooming standards, within reason. So it would be difficult, if not impossible, to pinpoint which haircuts and styles would or wouldn't enhance your career opportunities. Nevertheless, exercise judgment based on your own situation and some common sense: A thoroughly blown-out, spiky hairstyle that wins compliments for an art director, for example, would probably draw frowns and criticism at a Wall Street law firm. First establish how your hair must *perform* to work within the context of your lifestyle. *Then* turn your attention to aesthetic considerations.

This is the part where you might think I'm going to tell you that an oval face is wonderful, and if yours is round, you should do everything in your power to make it seem oval. But I won't, because I don't for a moment believe that.

After all, humankind boasts an incredible array of physical types. How can one shape or size be superior to another? Besides, what if your hair won't do precisely what it would have to do to make your face the "perfect" shape?

Granted, if you happen to have a long face supported by a long neck, you don't want to stretch the length any farther. And certainly most of us have some flaw that we'd at least like to hide—even if no one else ever noticed it. So what you should really want is not to change the shape of your face or to take some other equally drastic measures but rather to achieve a better proportion, the kind of balance that will flatter *the shape your face has* and to take attention away from a feature or features you dislike. Here are some guidelines to help you accomplish both with haircut and hairstyle:

- Hair cut very short or pulled back will highlight the shape of your face and your features. To minimize prominent features, consider a full hairstyle to bring more attention to your hair.
- If you have full cheeks or a round face, a bowl-shaped cut and styles that are wide at the sides will accentuate these characteristics. To diminish the roundness of your face, consider long hair cut at an angle or short hair worn somewhat close to the sides but with height and texture in the crown area.
- Full hairstyles, wide at the sides, on the other hand, tend to balance narrow faces.
- If your face is narrow and your forehead high, you may want to add bangs to shorten the effect a little more.
- Prominent noses do better with side parts because they tend to draw the eyes away from the centers of the faces.
- Bangs cut straight across will make a square jawline look even squarer.
- Hairstyles with lift and volume at the temples tend to balance wide jawlines; to make a jawline seem even narrower, try a chin-length cut styled closely to your face.
- To divert attention away from your chin entirely, keep your hair well below chin length—or above it. Shorter hairstyles with lots of texture in the crown are a good way to accomplish this.
- Do you want to bring attention to your eyes? You can do so with waves or curls near the temples, with wispy bangs swept to the side, or with longish bangs cut straight across. (If you have a small forehead, you can start your bangs fairly well behind the hairline.)

These hints may or may not help give you the "perfect" face according to some standards, and remember you also can use makeup to advantage. But with some thoughtful planning, they'll net you a high performance cut that does justice to the fabulous face you have and the beautiful hair that frames it.

SEVEN

HAIR DESIGNS: LOOK LIKE A WINNER YOUR WAY!

Conventional wisdom holds that successful management of your hair is all in the cut. While that popular idea may reflect a glimmer of truth (not to mention the responsibility it lays on the hairdresser), even a fabulous cut can flop miserably unless you know how to use it to change your hairstyle quickly and efficiently. For no matter how good it looks, wet or in its natural dry state, hair worn only one way is a lot less successful than hair you can vary to suit your mood and the occasion.

To illustrate, I have chosen a number of sports celebrities whose haircuts, and the style variations they can achieve with those cuts, demonstrate how this philosophy works in actual practice. Of course, the hairstyles photographed on these pages aren't the only options. With enough patience, these women could execute any number of hair designs that need a lot of fussing if they had the time.

But like you, they have jobs. For sportswomen that means globe-trotting virtually all year round to enter and win as many competitions as possible, not to mention training and personal appearances when they're not competing. Like you, they have home lives and responsibilities that must be met no matter how exhausted they may feel after stints in the outside world temporarily left behind. Like you, they have social commitments and other interests, apart from work and families, with little time to enjoy either.

And in order to maintain their good looks under the weight of all these demands, they need quick and easy approaches to hairstyling that require little thought or effort.

So, in this chapter, I'll show you examples of terrific-looking hairstyles for day and evening that fill this need. They're created with some of the styling techniques most of my clients have learned to use and can be achieved in almost no time flat because whenever possible, they utilize the hair's own tendency to bend or not to bend. (That includes what your hair wants to do after perming or relaxing.) And when it's not feasible to make use of the hair's own wave pattern (or absence of one), the hairstyle follows the line of least resistance to change, again making it fast and easy to create.

The hair designs featured on aerobics whiz Denise Austin and Olympic diver Jennifer Chandler (see photos on pages 63 and 64) provide good examples. In each case one version takes full advantage of the athlete's natural wave. Yet both women can alternate that with a smooth effect because their waves stretch readily with the help of a brush and blow-dryer, whereas curlier hair would resist stretching.

Basketball player Nancy Lieberman, whose evening look utilizes her perm in its most "natural" curly state, is another example. She also uses a round styling brush and blow-dryer to stretch her hair for one of the hair designs featured here (see photos on pages 81, 82). But Nancy wouldn't even attempt to get the kind of smoothness the other two can have.

I've included a variety of cuts and hair types for a good selection of styling techniques, some of which are bound to work for you. You may find you can borrow from one or from several to create a look uniquely your own. A few of the styles may seem difficult when you first read the instructions, but believe me, they're a lot easier to do than to explain in print. Obviously some hair, depending on thickness, may take a little longer to style. Nevertheless, all these hairdos can be executed quickly and easily—in record time, if need be. The trick is to develop a knack for the particular styling techniques that work best for you (all spelled out in Chapter 5). Some require no skill whatsoever. To "scrunch" your hair for added texture, for example, simply grasp a handful of hair and squeeze, crumpling it as you would paper. Repeat the process all over your head, or in specific areas, such as the ends or the crown, depending on the look you want to achieve. With a little practice, even more complex maneuvers will become second nature to you.

All the hairstyles call for a mousse or a gel applied to wet hair immediately after shampooing. No matter what kind of hair you have or which product you use to give it that extra boost, always work it first into the temples, then up through the crown area, where almost everyone needs the most help.

Each set of step-by-step styling instructions lists the implements needed and the kind of hair and cut on which it was created.

JENNIFER CHANDLER

HAIR: medium-textured, wavy and long, cut to all one length.

STYLING AIDS: gel; blow-dryer; plastic-quill brush.

METHOD:

- Apply gel to wet hair.
- With head pitched downward, blow-dry at medium setting. As hair dries, slide fingers through, from root area, gently pulling hair away from your scalp.
- Periodically scrunch the ends to get as much texture as possible into your loose waves.
- Then toss your hair back, and with the plastic-quill brush, work the temples and the front hairline sections for volume and lift (see instructions for this maneuver in Chapter 5).

  To smooth this hairstyle for variety, add a round styling brush, a plastic spray bottle of water, and hair spray.
- Spray your hair with a fine mist of water, then drop your head forward, and, with your dryer on high speed, use your plastic-quill brush to blow out all the curl and wave.
- Then wrap the ends of your hair around your styling brush, and apply some heat from your dryer, gently pulling the brush through, leaving those ends with a soft curve.
- If your hair needs more lift and volume (it might, after all that handling), back-comb at the temples (see instructions in Chapter 5).
- Finally, add some hair spray at the crown and temple areas, holding the hair upright away from the scalp, and blow-dry for a few seconds on a low setting.

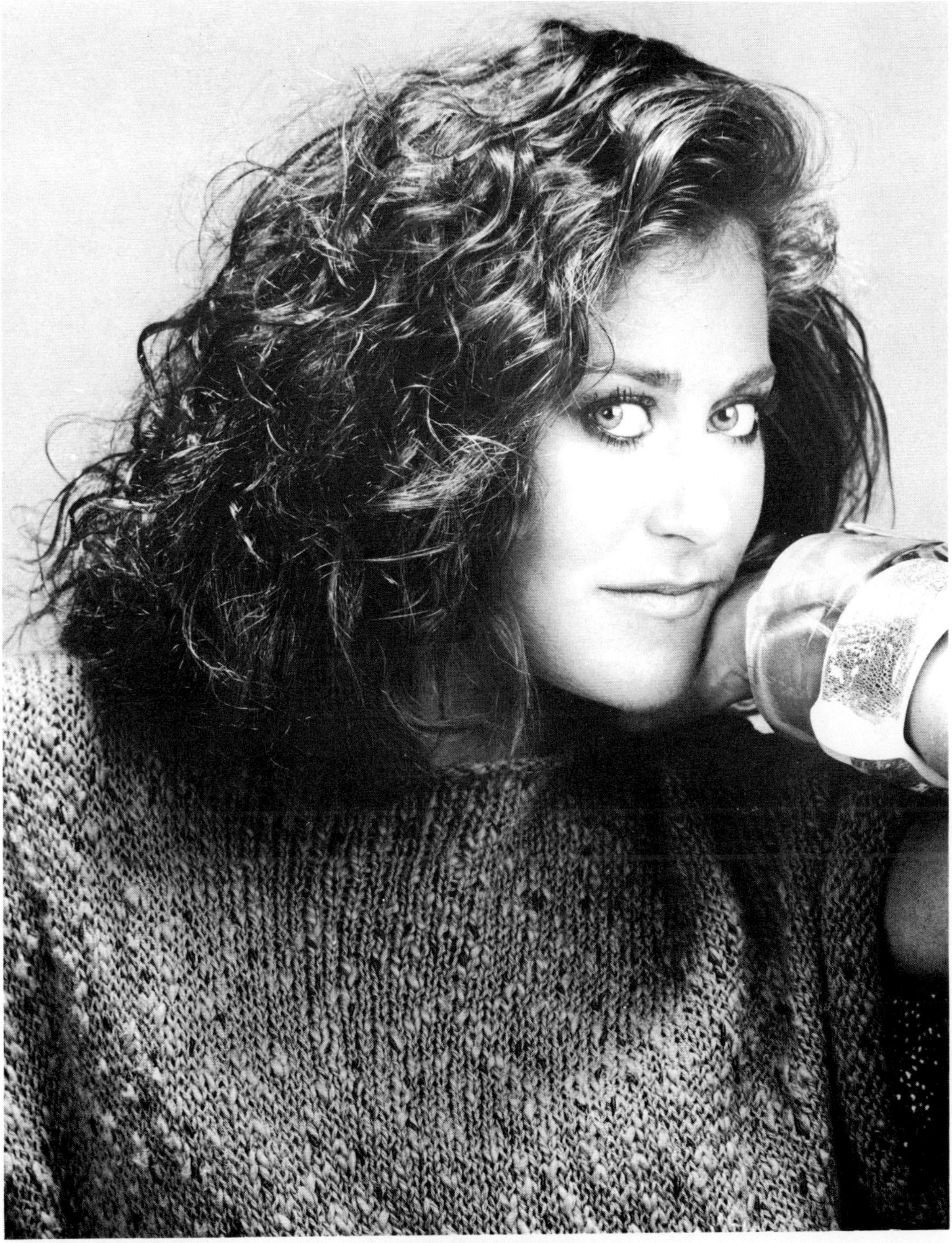

JENNIFER CHANDLER

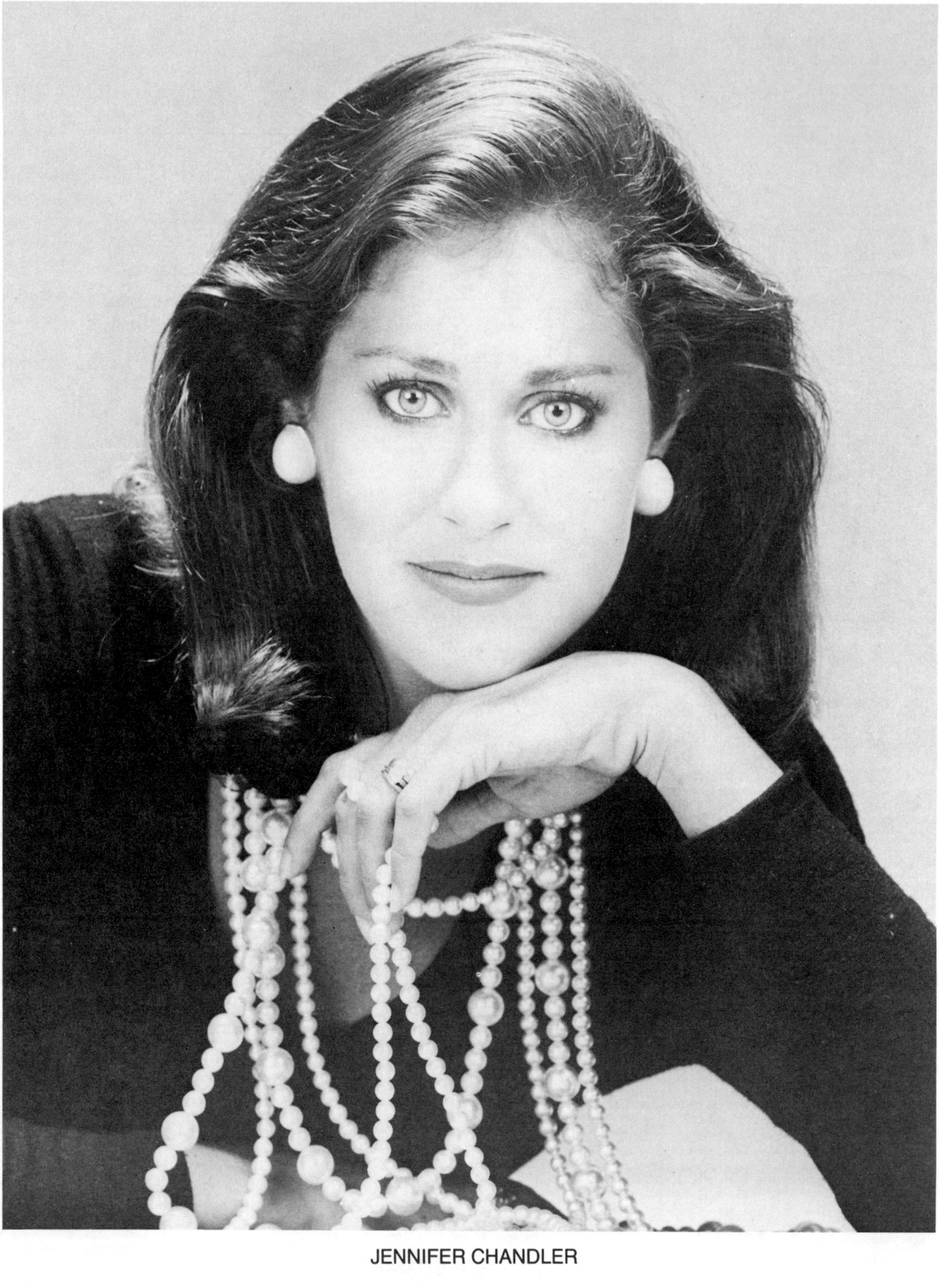

JENNIFER CHANDLER

JUDY BLUMBERG

HAIR: medium-textured with a strong wave, cut short and layered; highlights enhance texture and show movement.

STYLING AIDS: mousse; blow-dryer.

METHOD:

- Apply mousse to wet hair.
- Direct hair back through the top and temples with fingers, lifting upward for volume, and at the same time, blow-dry at a medium setting.
- Repeat at back and nape, directing the hair inward from each side, toward the center of the head, following the curve of the napeline. (The hair will hug the head in a smooth line at the back and nape.)

To vary this style for a sleeker look, add some hair spray at the temples, sides, and back. Then, with a vented brush, diminish the volume at the sides and at the back portion of the crown, placing emphasis toward the front.

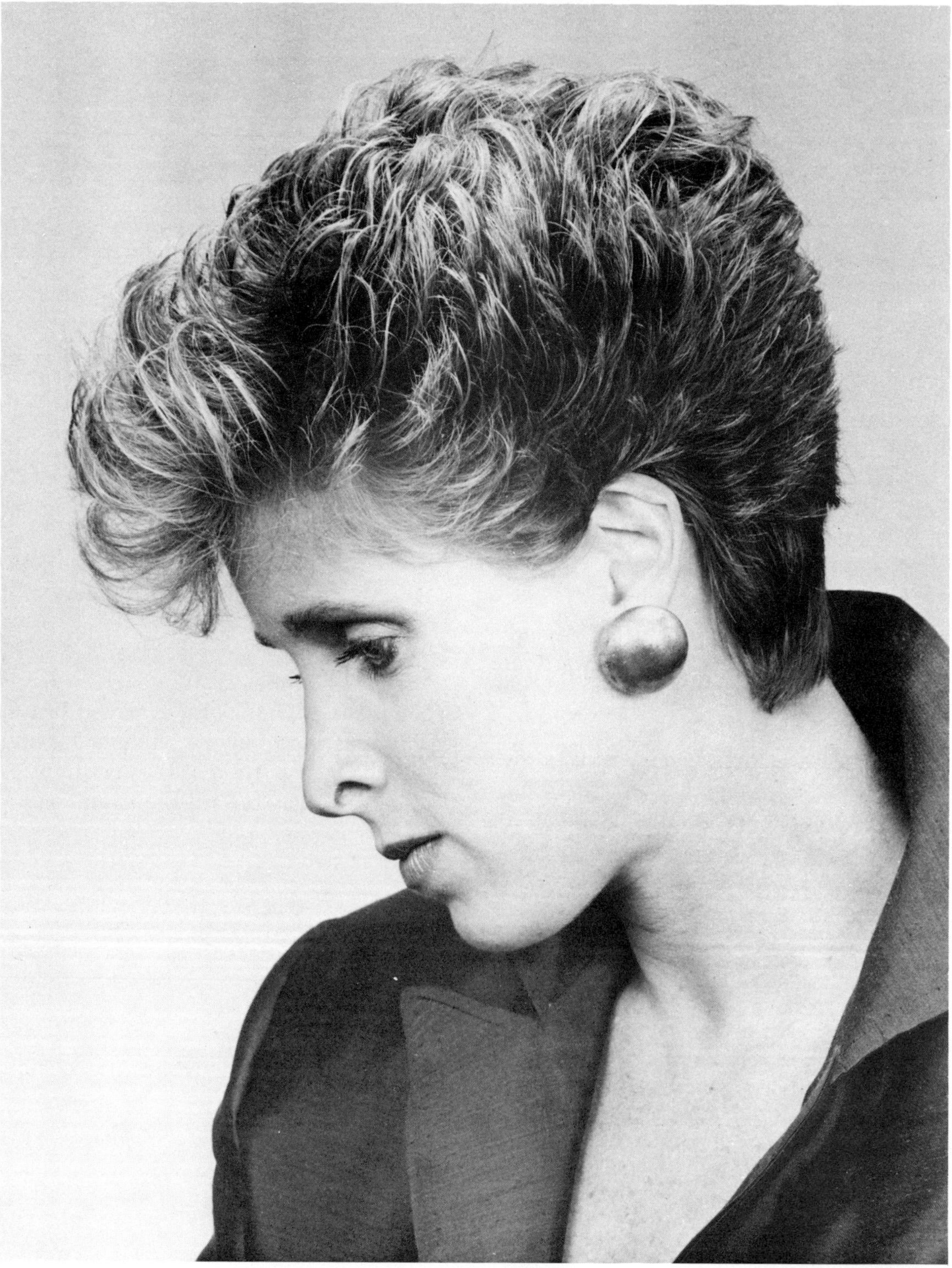

JUDY BLUMBERG

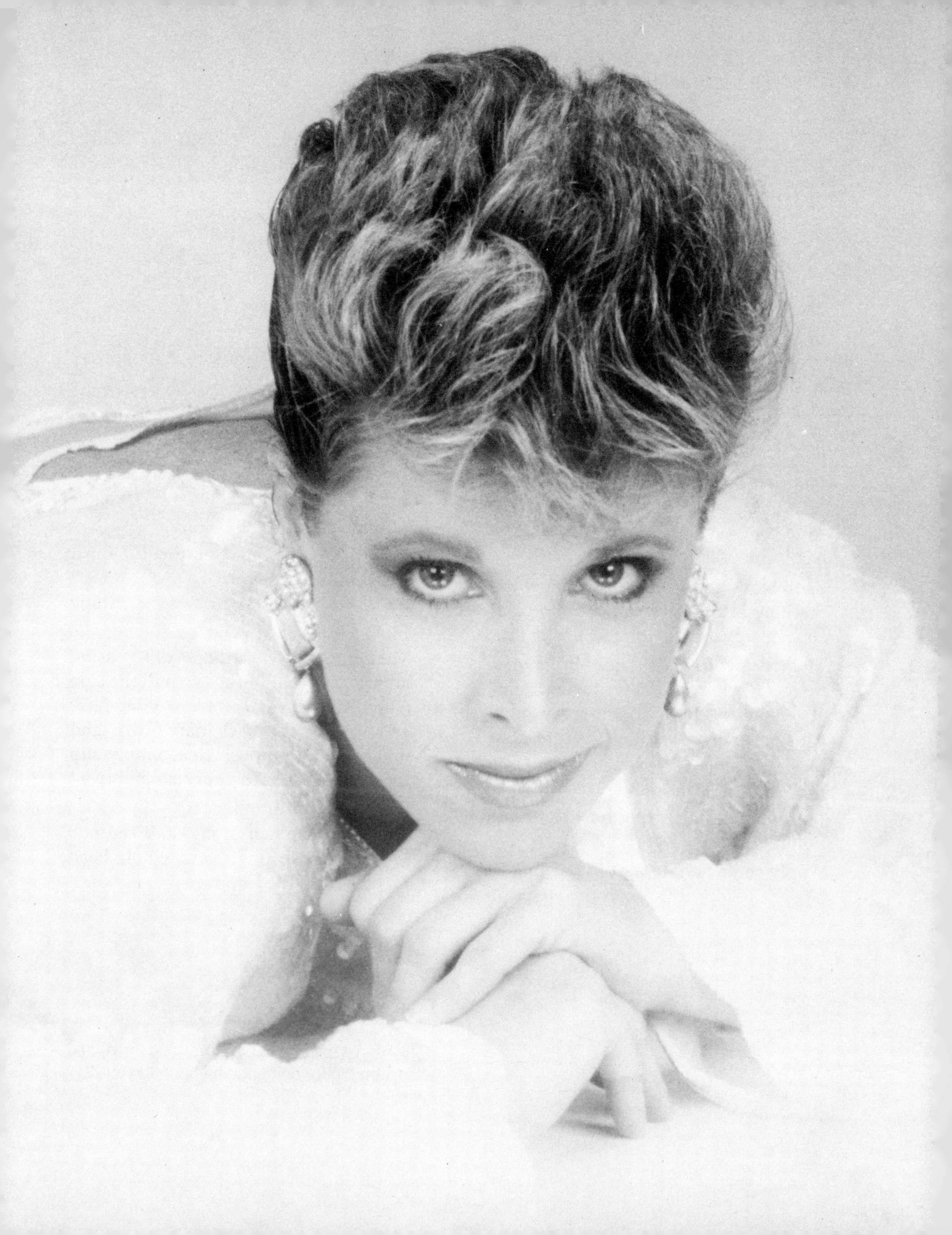

APRIL ALLEN

HAIR: medium-textured, straight with body wave and highlights, cut short and to all one length with some front layering.

STYLING AIDS: mousse; hair spray; blow-dryer; plastic-quill brush.

METHOD:

- Apply mousse to wet hair.
- With blow-dryer set on high, blow everything at the back upward. Force of air helps push hair up and dry it fast.
- Then, use your plastic-quill brush maneuver (see Chapter 5 for instructions) at temples with dryer still set at high; lift your hair up and away from your face.
- Use the same maneuver at the front on top, this time lifting for height and volume.
- Apply some hair spray to your fingertips, and work it through the wisps all around the face and at the sideburn areas, pulling forward.

For the variation, you need a plastic spray bottle of water.

- Mist the sides and back only, using your plastic-quill brush to pull the side hair forward, more toward your face, and to pull the back hair down and under. To accomplish this, simply slip the quill brush into your hair and twist in a downward motion.
- Apply a little hair spray, and scrunch your fingers through your whole head of hair for added texture.

April Allen's hair, shown before (see inset) and after perming for body and highlighting for richness.

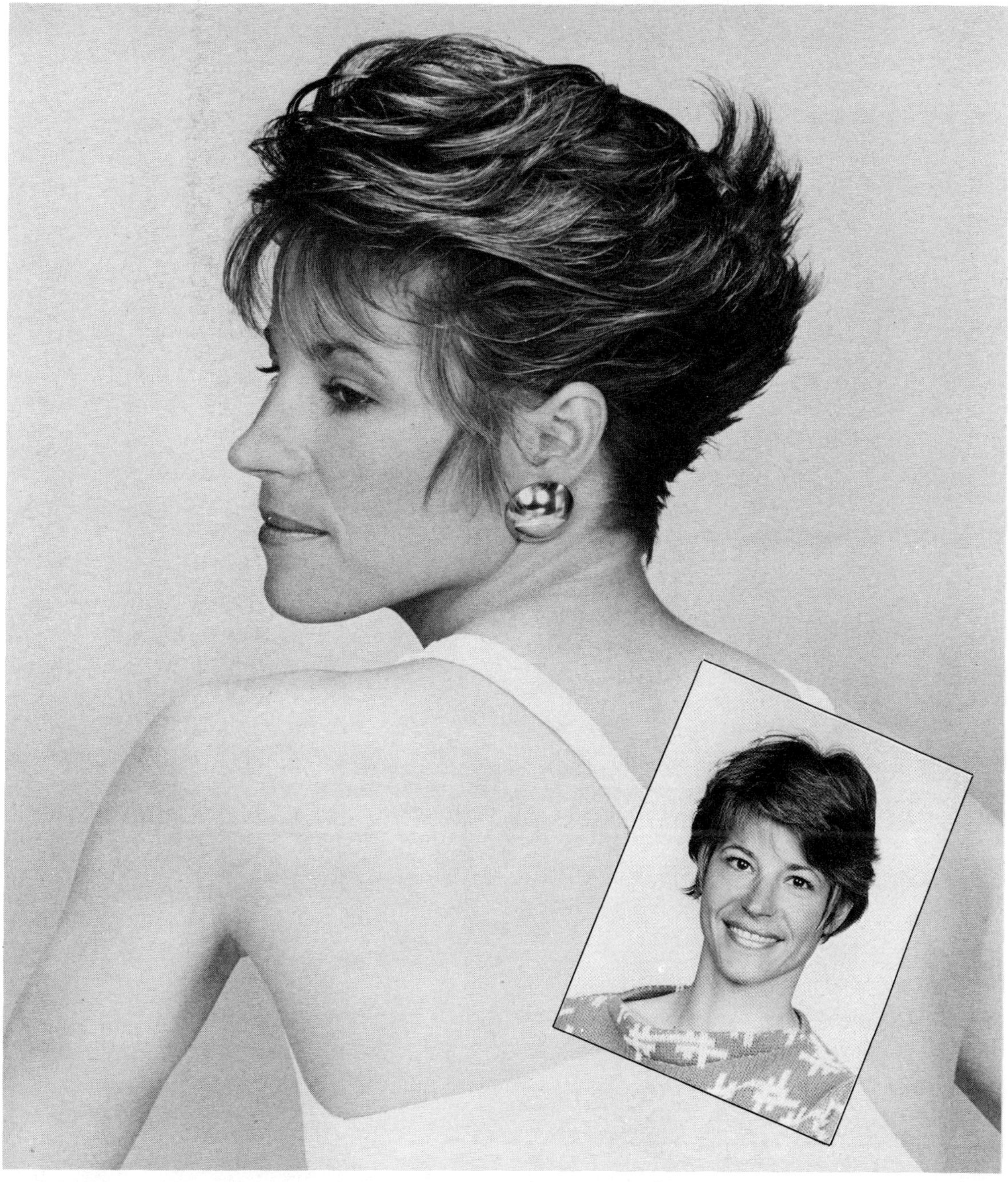

APRIL ALLEN

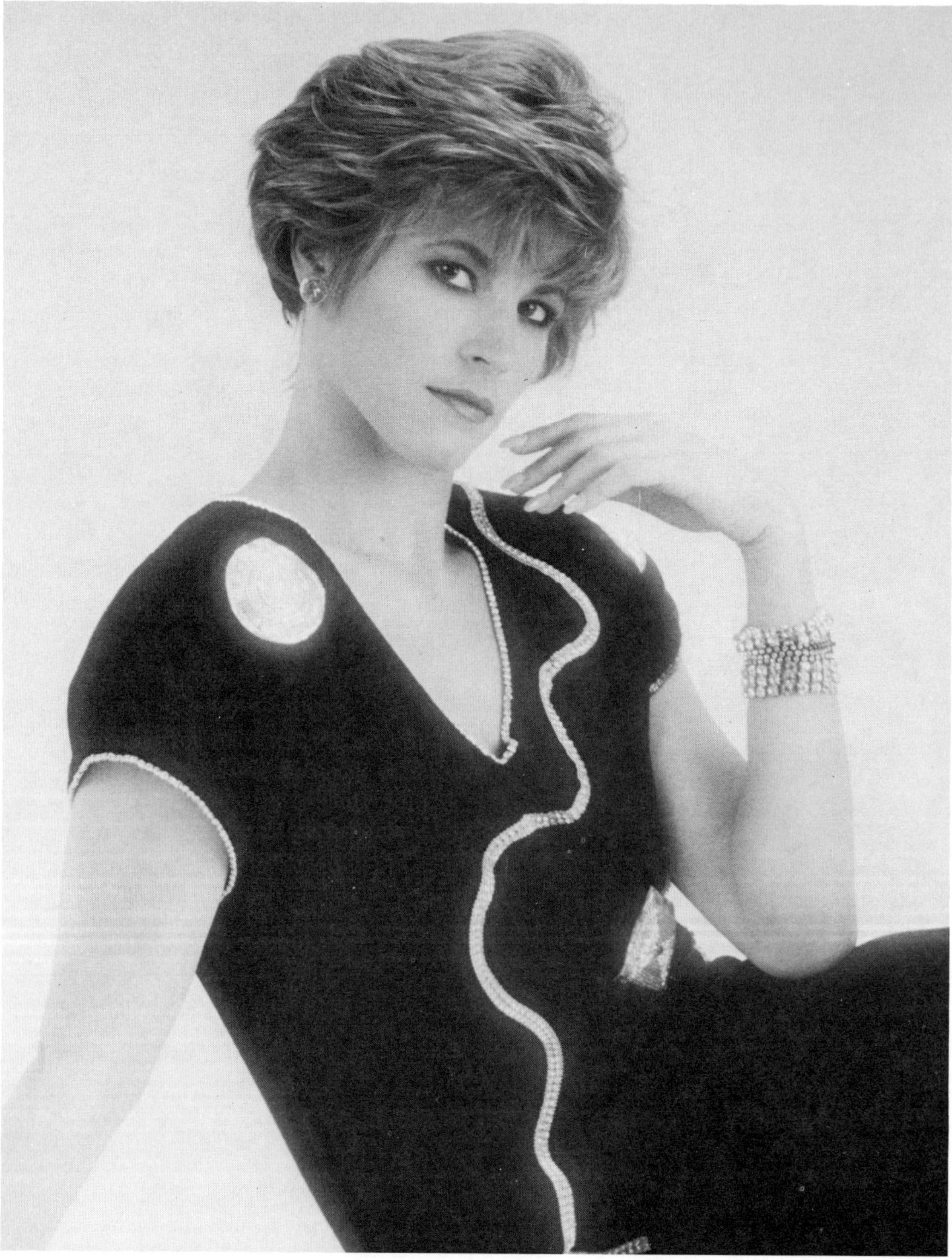

APRIL ALLEN

MARTINA NAVRATILOVA

HAIR: finely-textured, cut to medium length and layered, tinted blond.

STYLING AIDS: mousse; hair spray; blow-dryer; plastic-quill brush; round styling brush.

METHOD:

- Apply mousse to wet hair.
- Throw your head forward, and blow-dry on high speed, using your plastic-quill brush to guide all the hair toward the crown and the crown hair away from the scalp.
- When your hair is about eighty-five percent dry, place head upright, and use your plastic-quill brush to get the layers to lift some more and bend under. To do so, slide the brush into your hair, and twist forward (in this motion, your thumb moves in toward the back and the rest of your knuckles come forward).
- When hair is completely dry, use your round styling brush to increase the curve all around your face. Wrap the perimeter hair around the brush, winding it under.
- Do the same at the crown if you need more height there. Then spray with hair spray, and scrunch all over with fingers to get texture.

To vary the look, for a smoother evening style, you'll need a paddle brush and large hot rollers.

- Brush the hair to smooth it up and away from your face. Then place a large heated roller at each temple, rolled back at an angle. (If you need additional heated rollers in the back, roll them under.)
- When you remove rollers, brush the hair into place with a paddle brush.

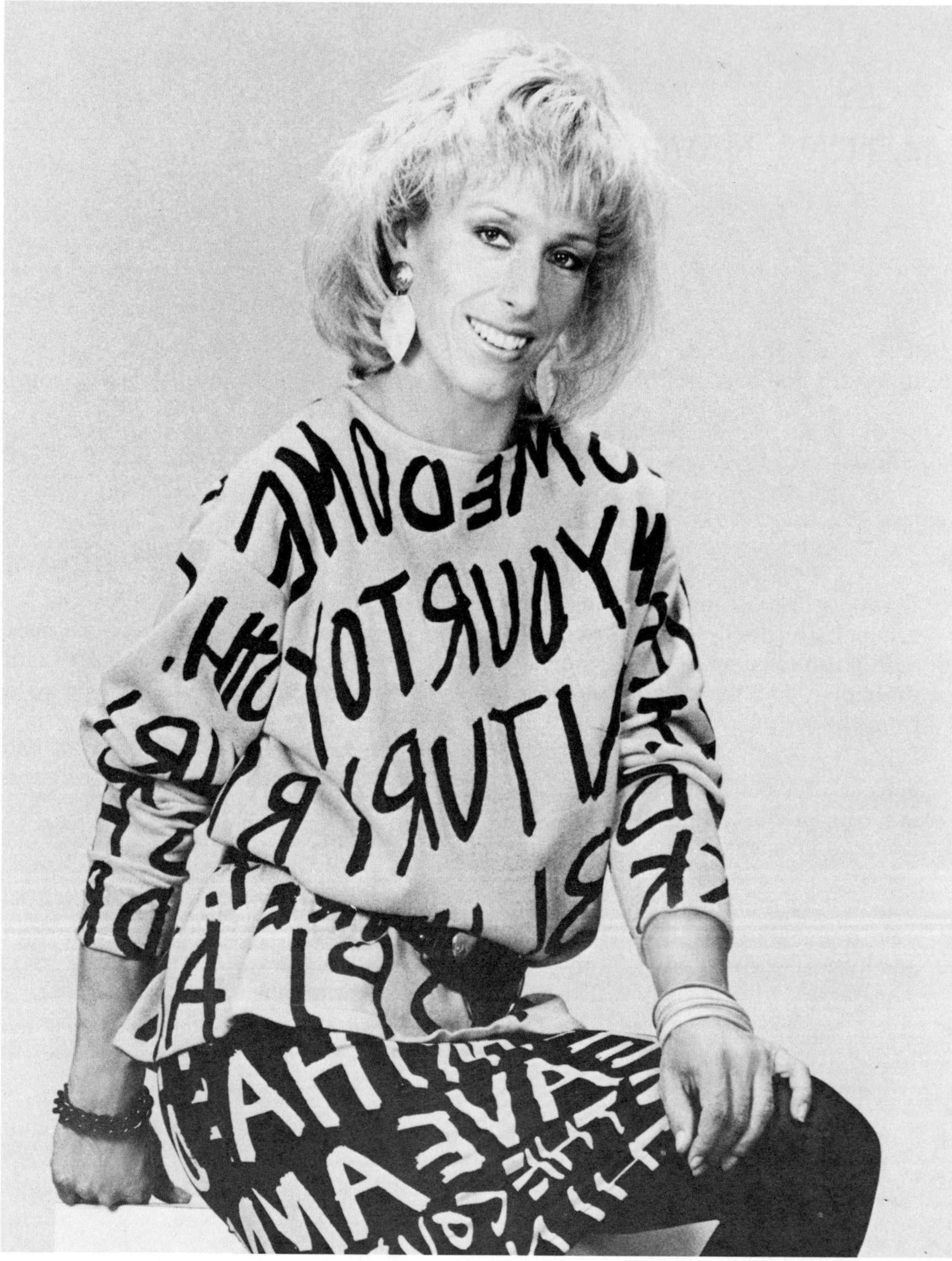

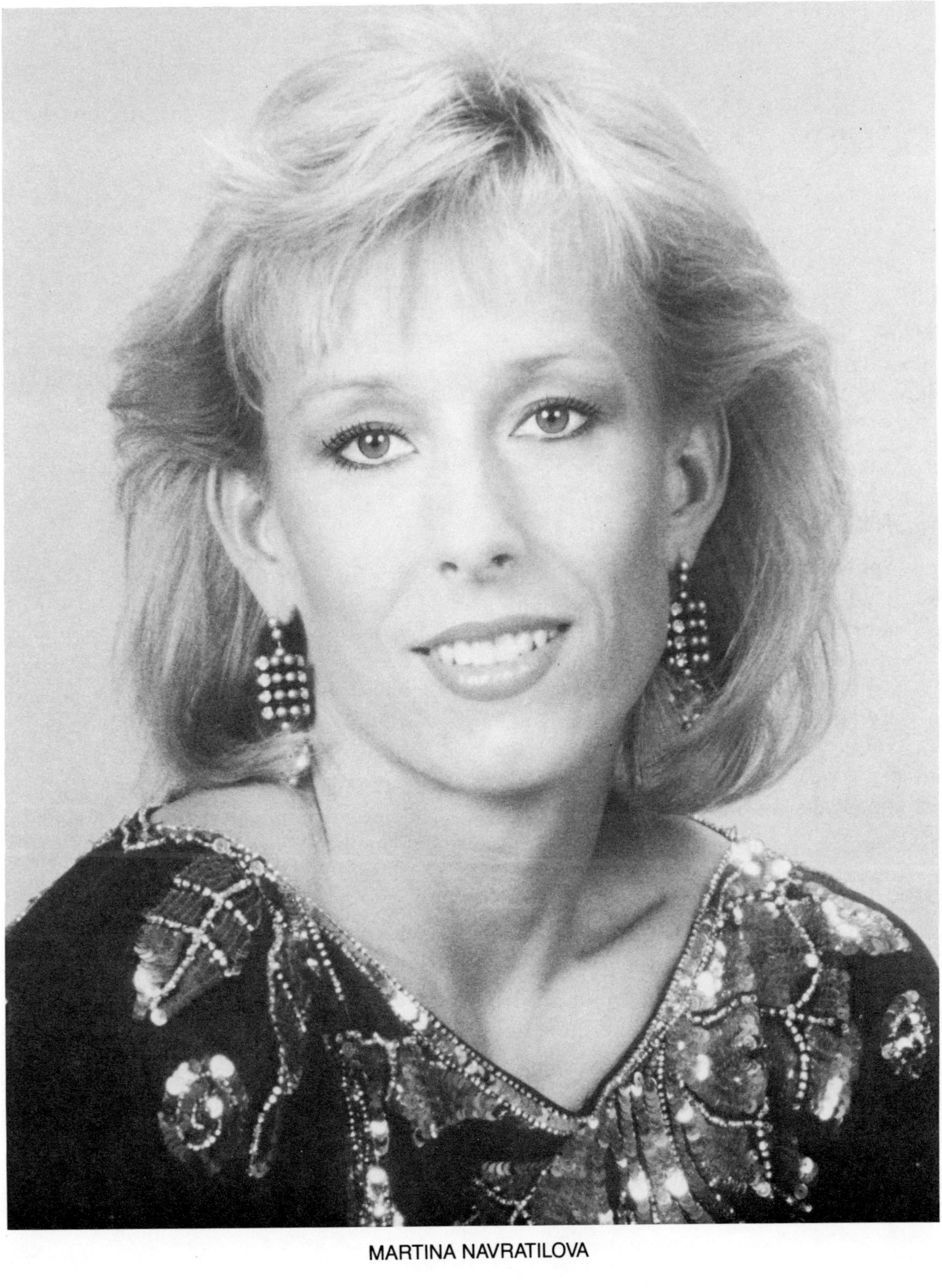

MARTINA NAVRATILOVA

DENISE AUSTIN

HAIR: medium-textured, wavy, abundant amount, cut to medium length, all one length with some layering around the face.

STYLING AIDS: mousse; hair spray; plastic-quill brush; round brush; blow-dryer.

METHOD:

- Apply mousse to wet hair.
- Bend your head forward, and with your blow-dryer on high setting, use your plastic-quill brush to stretch out virtually all the wave. As your hair is drying, gently tug hair away from your scalp.
- Place head upright, and continue smoothing the top areas.
- Use your round brush to curve the ends under, wrapping the hair around the brush and gently pulling the brush through the hair as you apply dryer heat.
- Afterward use your plastic-quill brush to put some lift and volume into the temple and crown sections (see Chapter 5 for step-by-step instructions).
- Finally, use your fingers to hold the top and temples away from your scalp. Add a touch of hair spray, and blow-dry for a second or two on a low setting.

To create a different look for evening, you need a plastic spray bottle of water, hair spray, a small paddle brush, and a pick-comb.

- Spray your hair with a fine mist of water. Then bend forward, and scrunch your hair all over with your fingers to bring back your natural wave and curl pattern.
- Place head upright, use your fingers to push the temple hair upward (see Chapter 5 for instructions), and hit the temple areas with a little hair spray.
- Then spray all over, and continue to scrunch your hair while it's still damp with hair spray. For more volume, backbrush with your small paddle brush, and use the pick-comb to place and lift where needed.

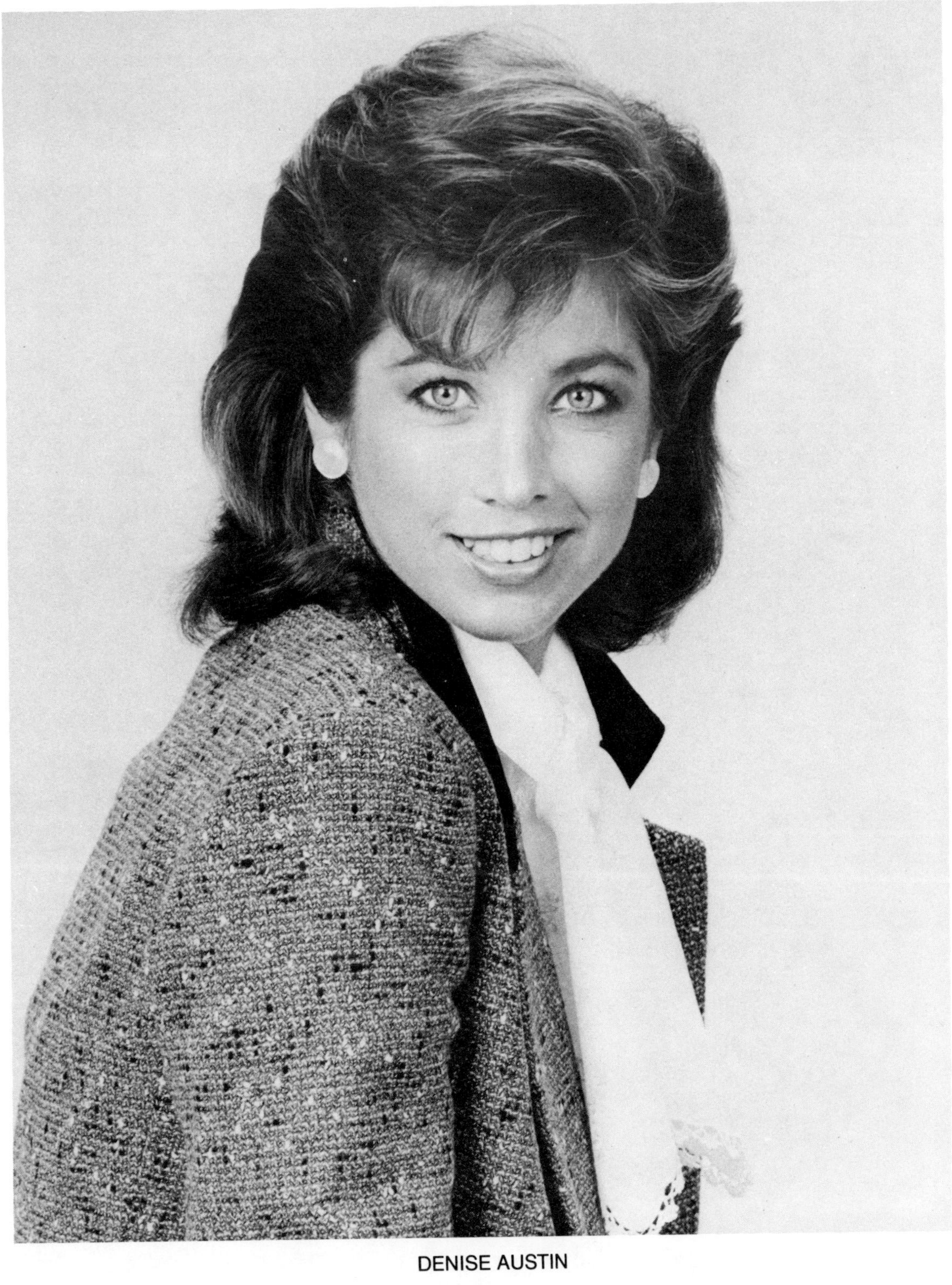

DENISE AUSTIN

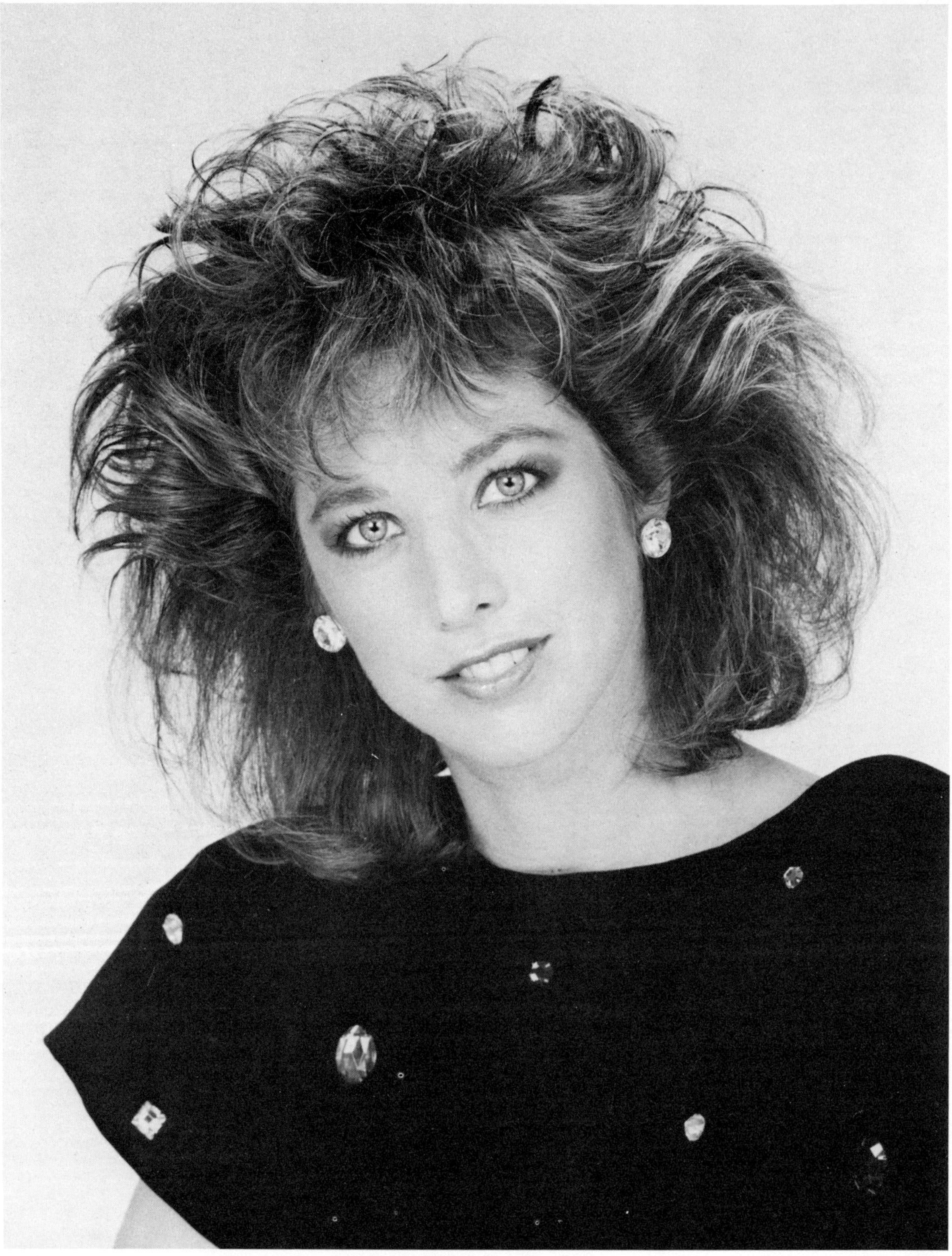

DENISE AUSTIN

DEBI THOMAS

HAIR: coarsely-textured, treated to relax curl, cut short in layers with some length at the back.

STYLING AIDS: gel; blow-dryer; plastic-quill brush.

METHOD:

- Apply gel to wet hair.
- Dry your hair at a high setting, using your plastic-quill brush to stretch and direct the hair, sweeping the temples upward and the front section toward one side.
- As you dry the back and nape areas, direct the hair downward by sliding your plastic-quill brush into the hair and twisting so your thumb rotates in toward your head and your other knuckles rotate away from your head. *To vary this look for dressier occasions,* add bobby pins, hairpins, and ornamental combs if desired.
- With your plastic-quill brush and your fingers, brush the hair from the left side of the nape area slightly up toward the right, and secure it with a row of bobby pins somewhat off center.
- Then sweep the hair from the right toward the left over the bobby pins, using your fingers to tuck in the ends, and secure with hairpins (and ornamental combs if you like), creating a French twist.
- Then spray the front section with a dash or two of hair spray, and scrunch the ends with your fingers for lots of texture.

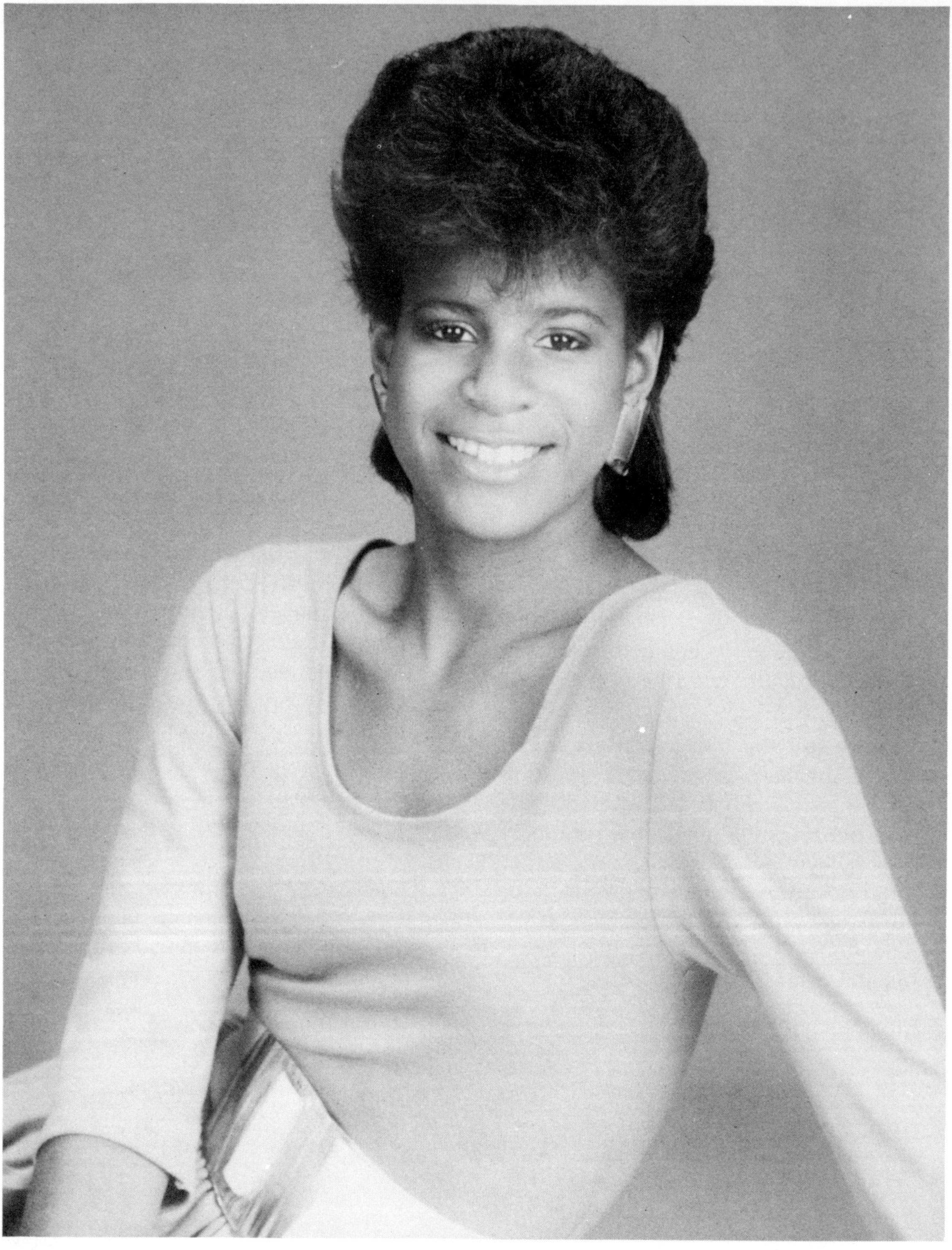

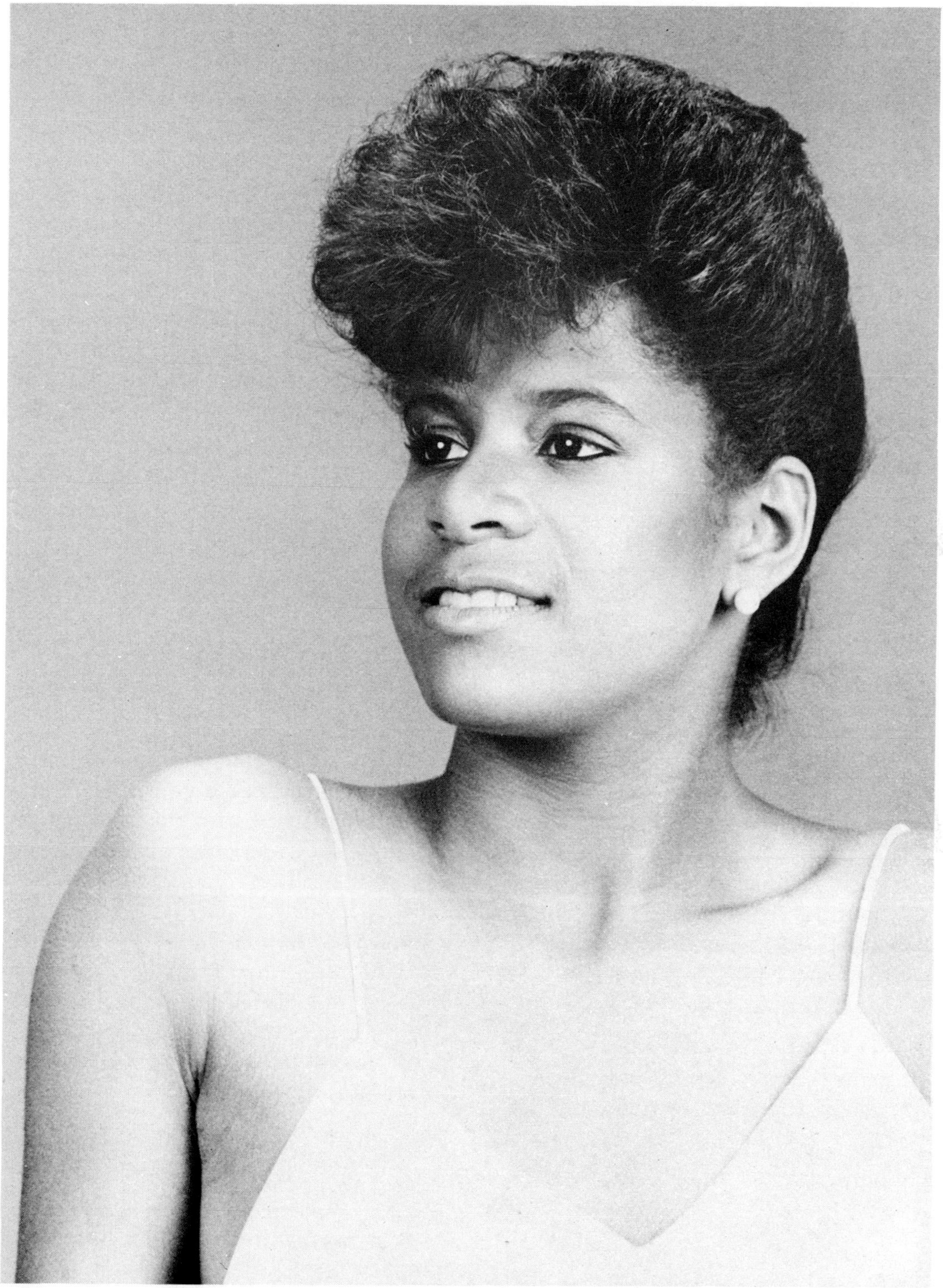

DEBI THOMAS

NANCY LIEBERMAN

HAIR: coarsely-textured, straight, and permed for body, with a short, layered cut.

STYLING AIDS: mousse; hair spray; blow-dryer; round styling brush; vented brush (optional).

METHOD:

- Apply mousse to wet hair.
- Throw your head forward. Dry quickly with blow-dryer on medium setting. Work your fingers through the hair as you're drying to get all the hair lifting, moving upward, stretching the curl pattern.
- When hair seems about eighty-five percent dry, place head upright, and finish with a round styling brush and blow-dryer at high speed, wrapping and stretching the sides and top, going toward the back, away from your face.
- The back goes under, following the same general direction, right down to the nape area.
- Using the styling brush and blow-dryer, wrap the front sections at the top, stretching the hair more toward the side, as you pull out the brush and apply heat.
- Then spray your fingers slightly, and pull a few wisps forward over your forehead.
- Finally, spray the sides and top with hair spray, and rake your fingers or a vented brush through your hair to get more texture and press the sides closer to your head.

  To vary this look for dressy occasions, simply spritz your head all over with a light mist of hair spray, and use your fingers to scrunch the hair. This will bring back all the texture, wave, and curl you stretched out with the blow-dryer and brush.

The inset shows Nancy's perm before styling, which works well for a curly look; the larger picture shows her perm styled with mousse and a blow dryer.

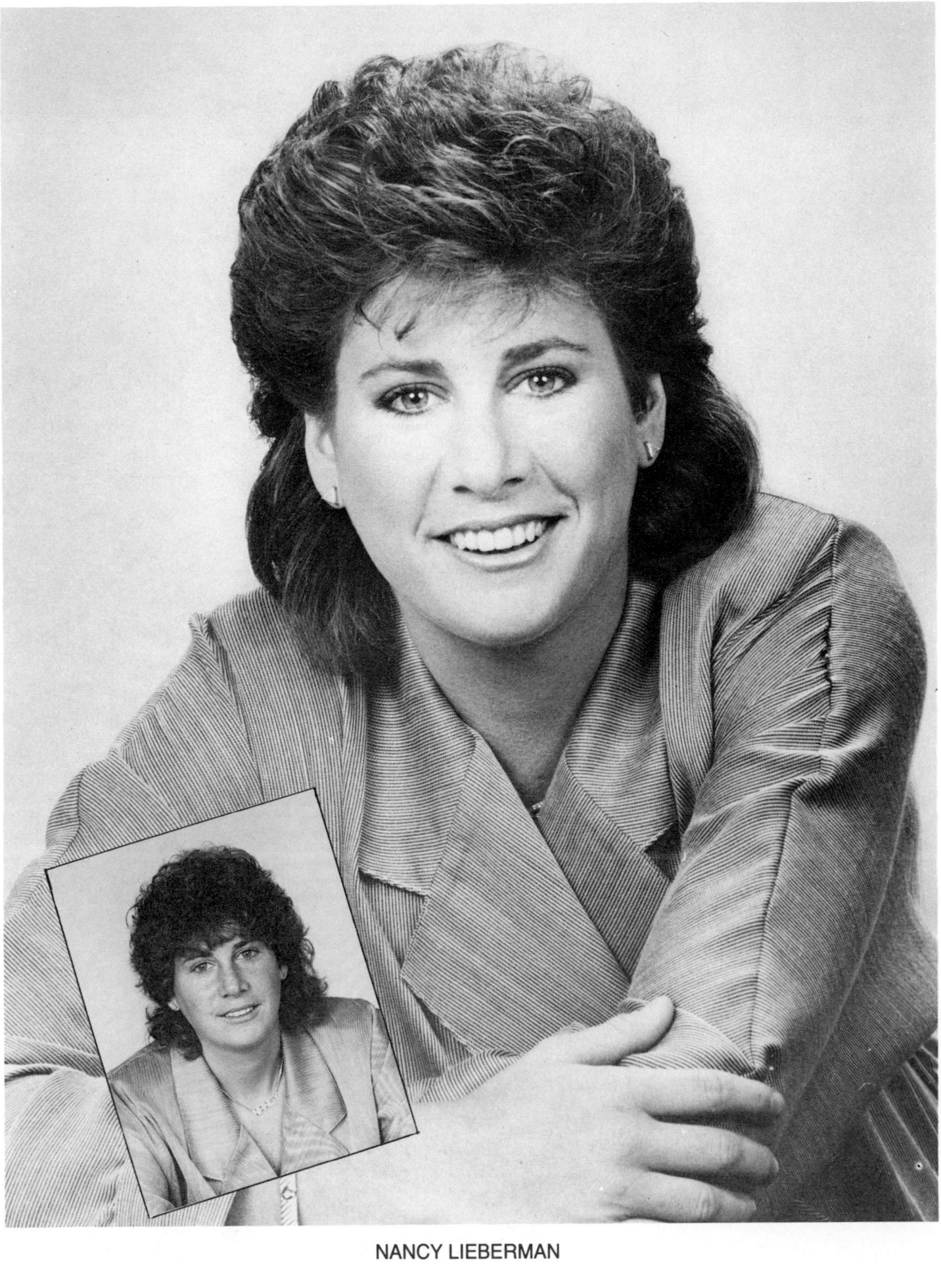

NANCY LIEBERMAN

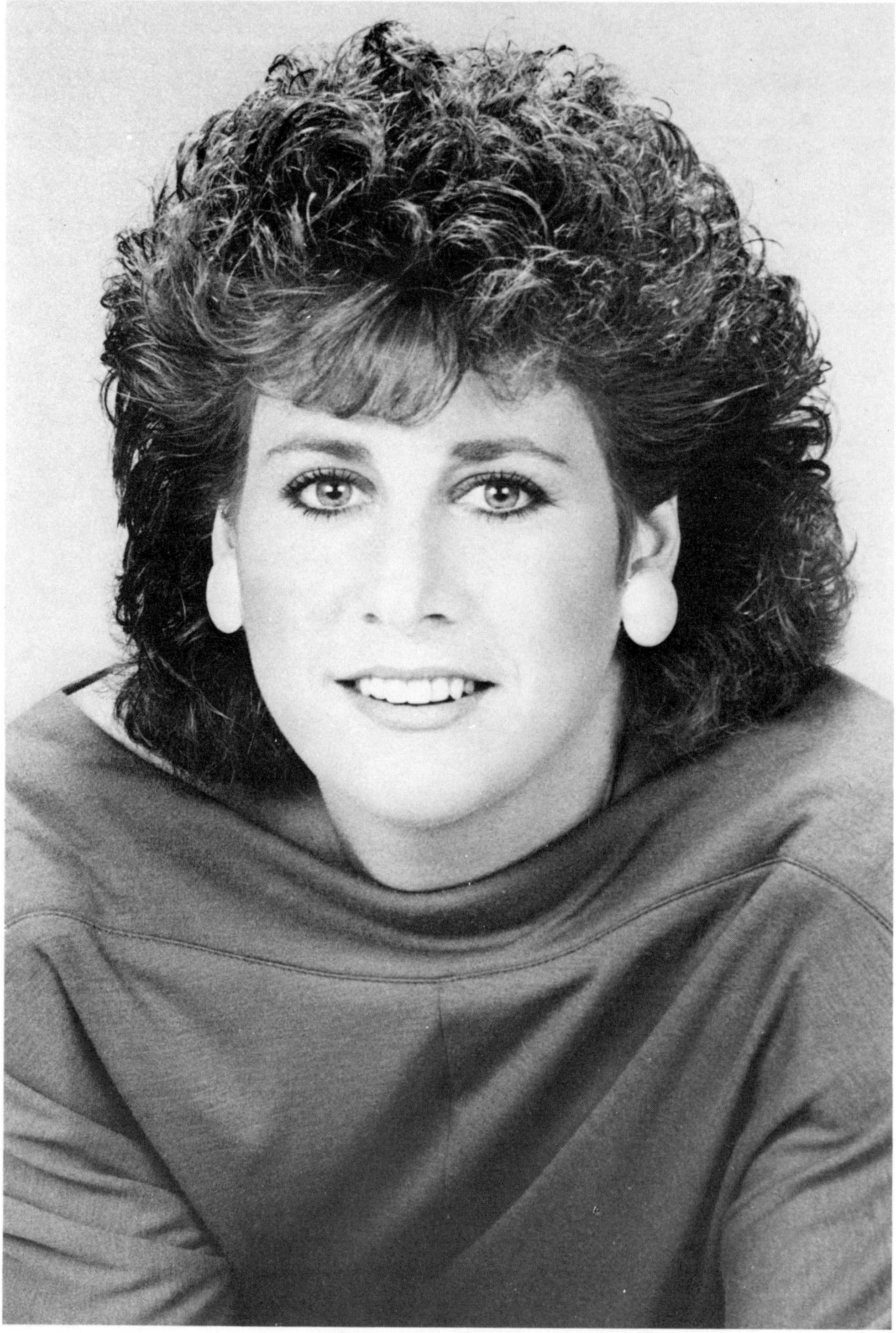

NANCY LIEBERMAN

GLADYS PORTUGUES

HAIR: coarsely-textured, curly, long, and layered.

STYLING AIDS: gel; plastic-quill brush; blow-dryer.

METHOD:

- Apply gel to wet hair.
- With head bent forward, blow-dry at medium setting, using your fingers and plastic-quill brush to direct the hair away from your scalp.
- When the hair is about eighty-five percent dry, flip it back, and use plastic-quill brush at temples to lift hair away from the face, in the crown for additional volume, and in the bang area for direction (see Chapter 5 for step-by-step instructions for this maneuver).
- Finish with a light, all-over touch of hair spray; then scrunch the outer sections (the ends) to give curls more definition.

To vary this look for evening, apply more mousse or gel to the temples, and get a large paddle brush.

- Use the brush to smooth all your hair into one ponytail, leaving the bangs undisturbed.
- Add a touch of hair spray for additional control, and adorn the ponytail with a length of lace, as Gladys did, or with some other festive ornament.
- If needed, use the plastic-quill brush once more on your bangs to give them more definition and lift.

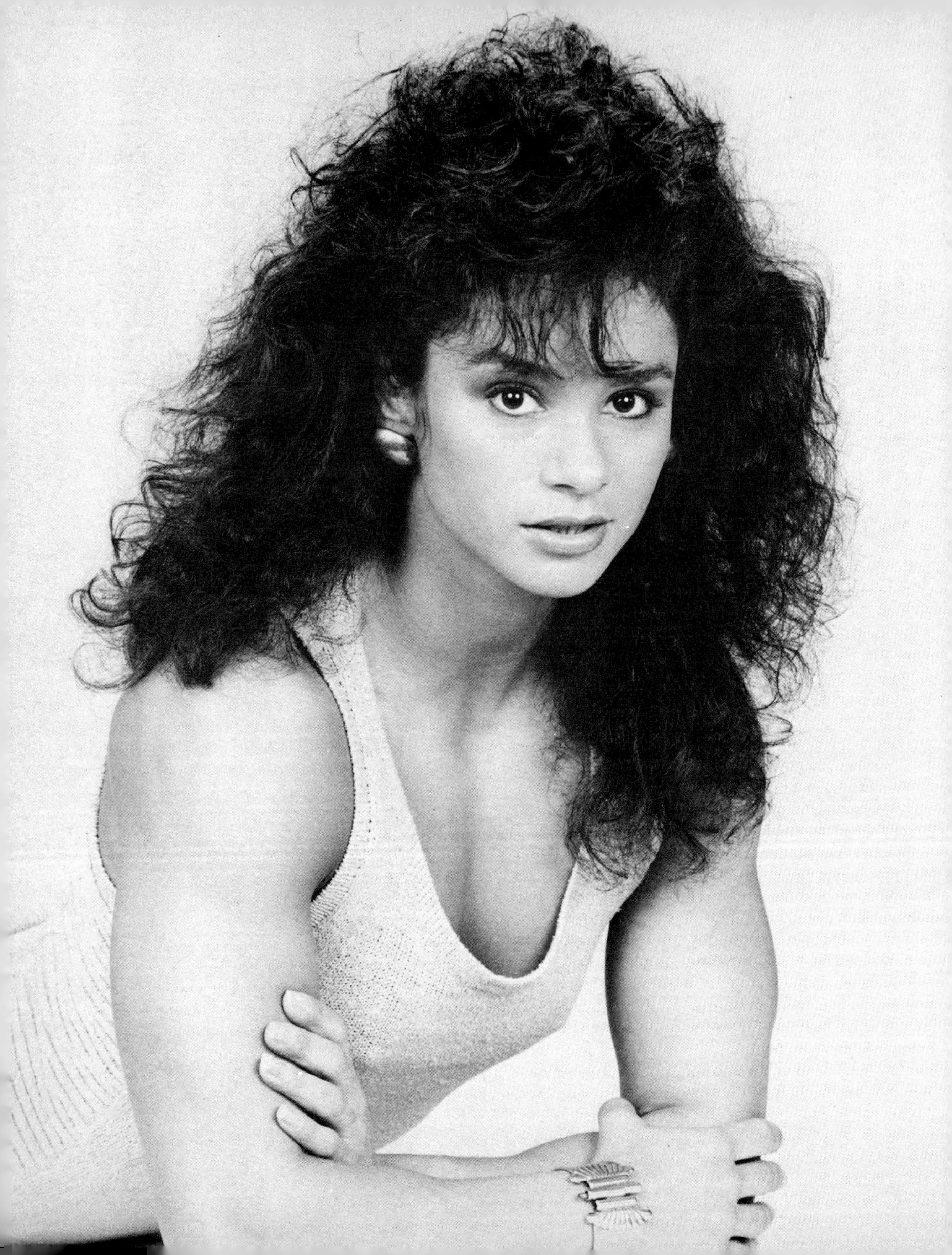

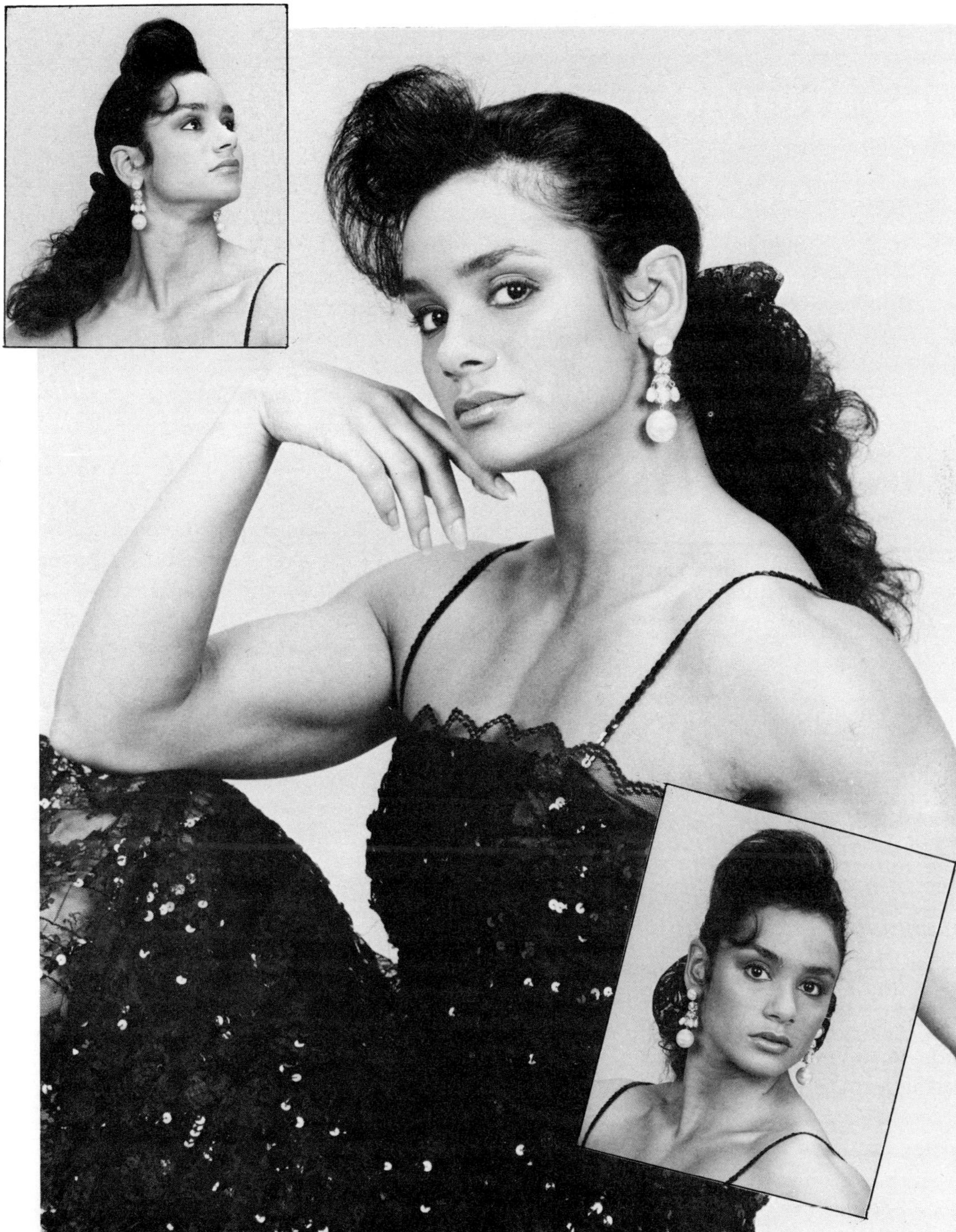

Gladys Portugues shows off her simple evening hairdo.

CHRIS EVERT LLOYD

HAIR: finely-textured, cut to medium-length and layered, permed, and highlighted.

STYLING AIDS: mousse; blow-dryer; curling iron; vented brush (optional).

METHOD:

- Apply mousse to wet hair.
- Keeping your head upright, use your blow-dryer at medium speed to dry your temples, pushing hair in an upward direction with your fingers (for the moment, don't worry about drying the ends at all). When one temple is dried, apply some hair spray. Repeat the drying process, always pushing the hair upward, on the other side; then hit it with hair spray, and throw your head forward to complete drying all the way to the ends. Constantly use your fingers to push all the hair away from the scalp. Pay extra attention to lifting and stretching your crown hair to ensure maximum volume on top.
- With hair completely dry, place your head upright, and spot-touch the ends with a curling iron—or leave the ends as they are for a spiky look.
- Then run your fingers through your hair to break up the curl, spray all over with hair spray, and scrunch the ends with your fingers.

  For a dressier evening look, use a round styling brush and blow-dryer to stretch the hair out from scrunchy to smooth.
- Smooth the temples up and away from your face, curl the hair on top back and the back hair under, always stretching with the brush and dryer.
- Then spray the temple on one side, and use your fingers or a vented brush to make the hair hug your head for a sleeker look. Repeat the process on the other side.
- Finally, spritz the top with hair spray, and work your fingers through that section for more texture and to pull a few wisps down onto your forehead.

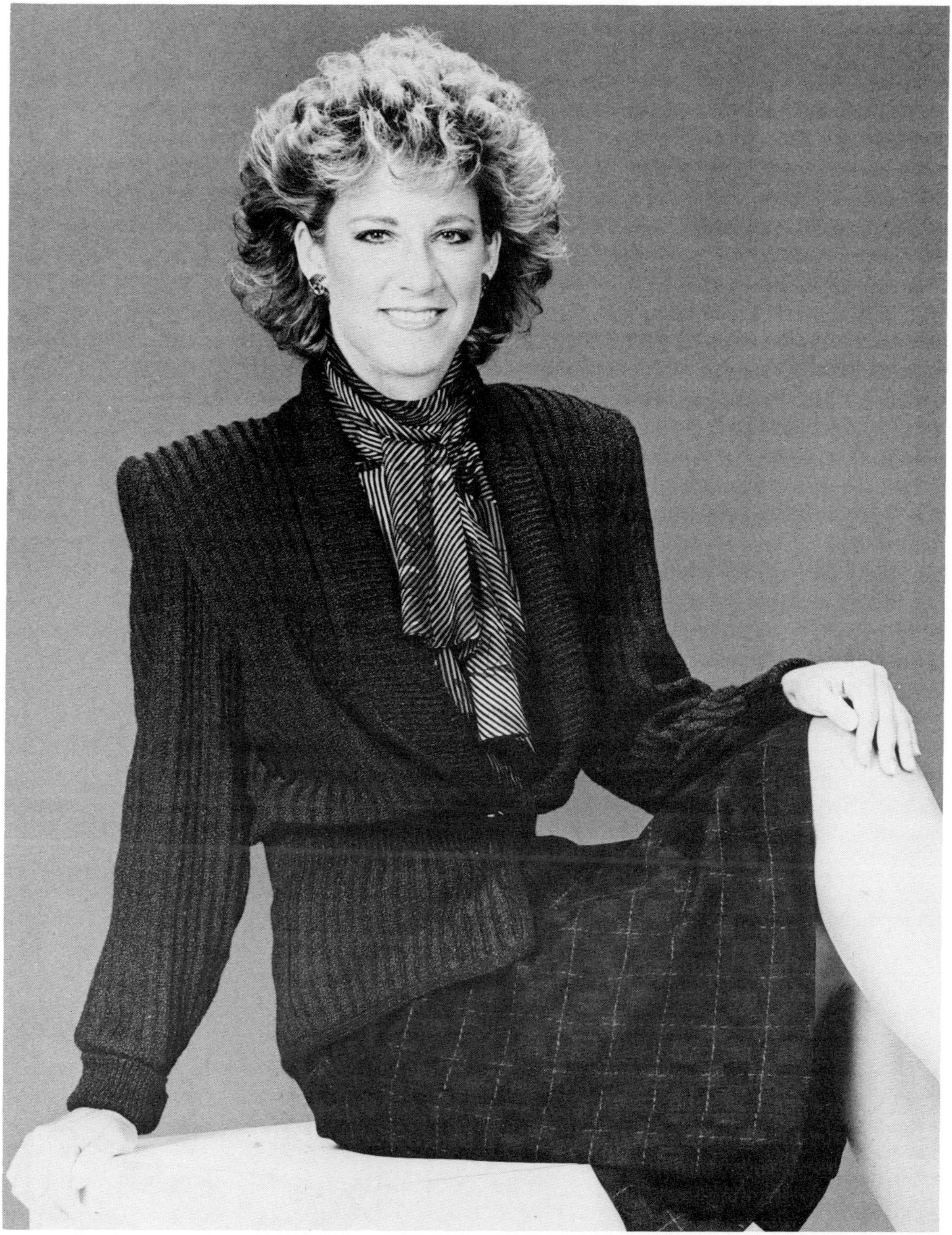

CHRIS EVERT LLOYD

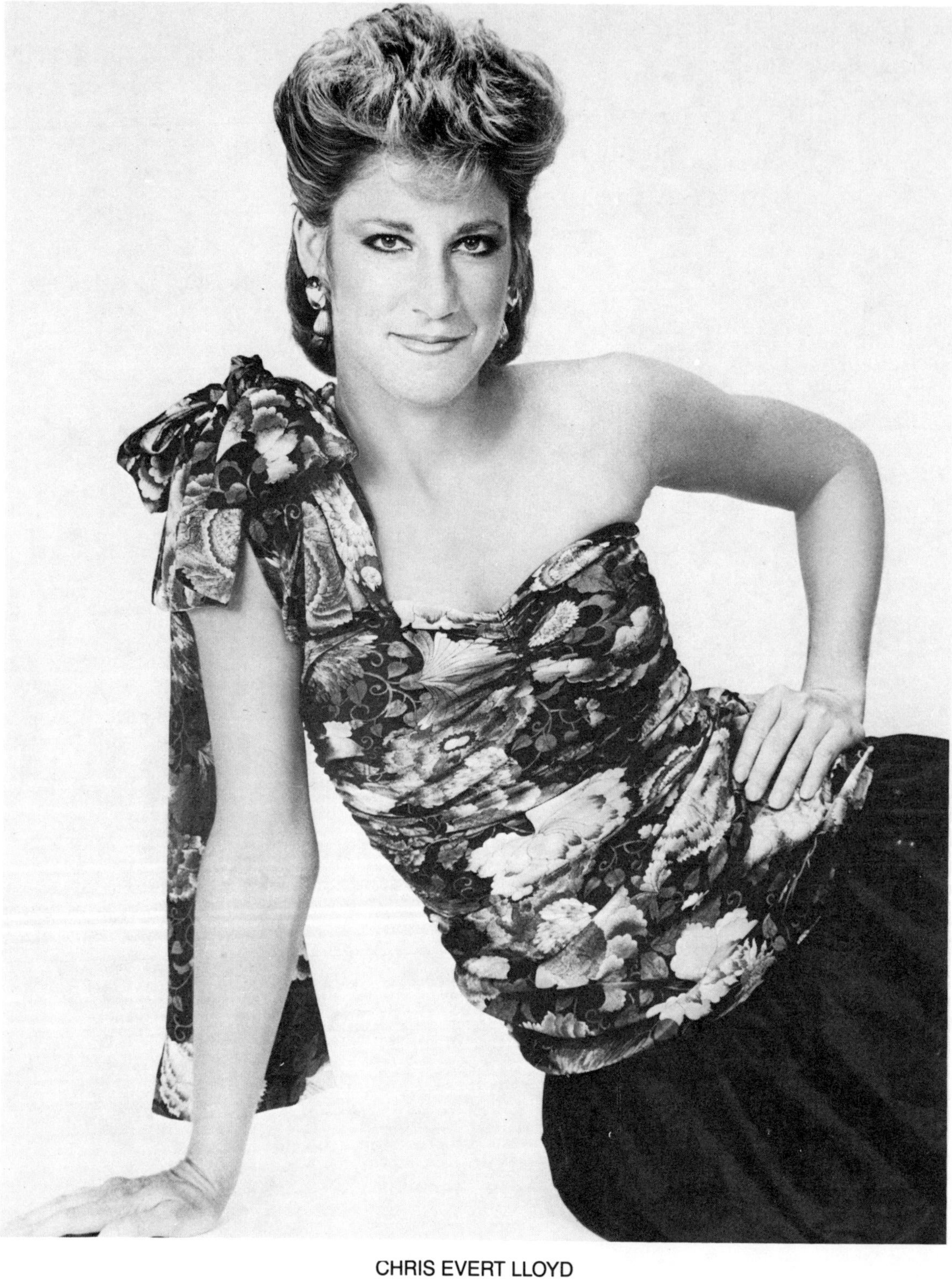

CHRIS EVERT LLOYD

HOLLIS STACY

HAIR: medium- to finely-textured, straight, cut in short layers.

STYLING AIDS: mousse; blow-dryer; hair spray.

METHOD:

- Apply mousse to wet hair.
- Slide fingers through hair, gently holding root areas away from scalp.
- Dry all the hair, holding it as above between the fingers, with the blow-dryer on a medium setting.
- From the nape area, move fingers up through the back toward the crown as you blow-dry to create volume.
- Finally, with a small amount of hair spray on your fingertips, direct forehead wisps down toward the face for more definition.

  To vary this look for evening, get a vented brush and a plastic spray bottle of water.
- Spray hair with a light, fine mist of water. Then rake your vented brush through the front, blending the wisps back into the hairstyle and through the rest of the hair for a sleek look that still has a lot of texture.
- Finally, for extra hold, add a light blast with hair spray, and dry in place with blow-dryer on low speed. (This time be sure to keep it still, rather than move it around, with the nozzle pointed specifically in the direction of your hairstyle.)

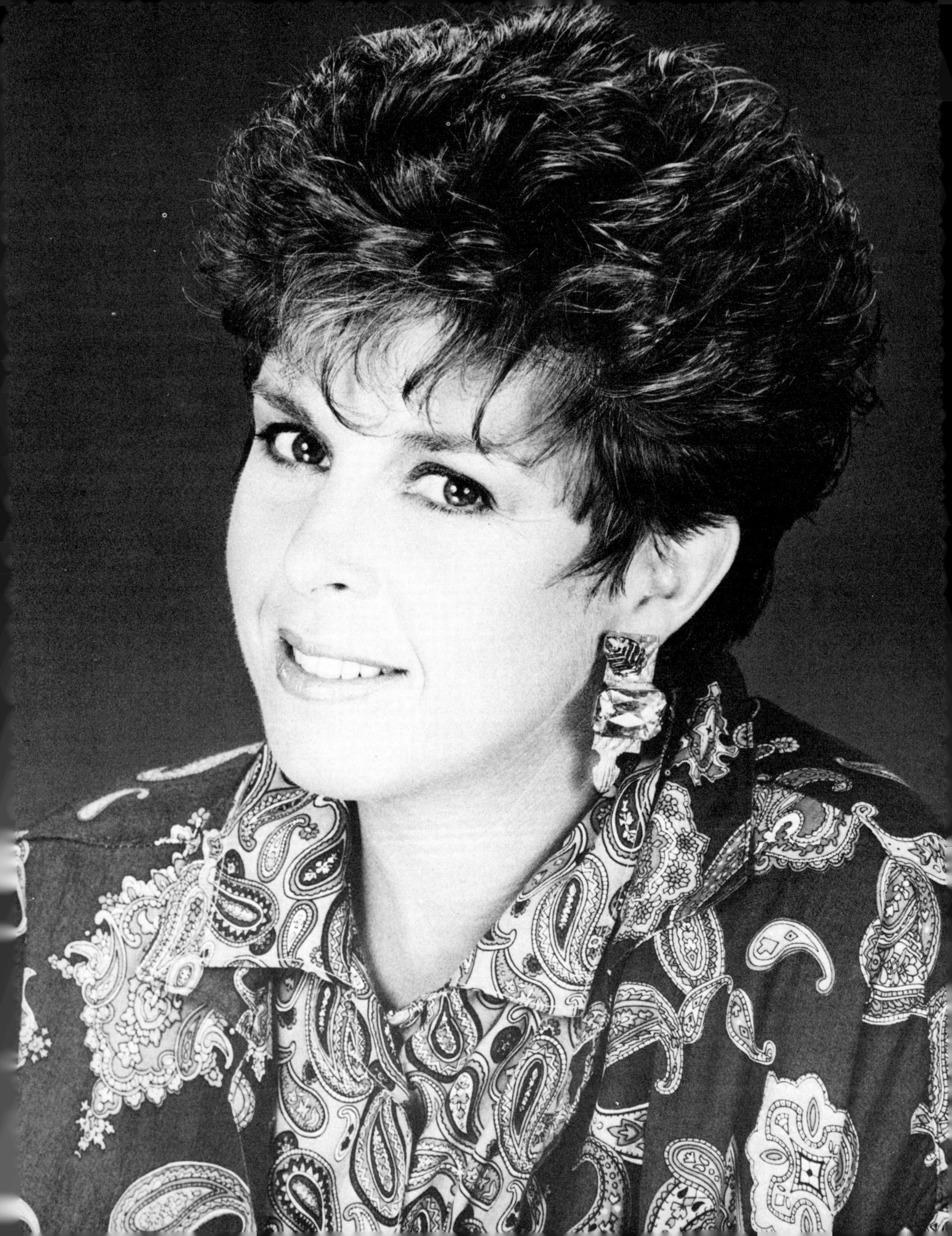

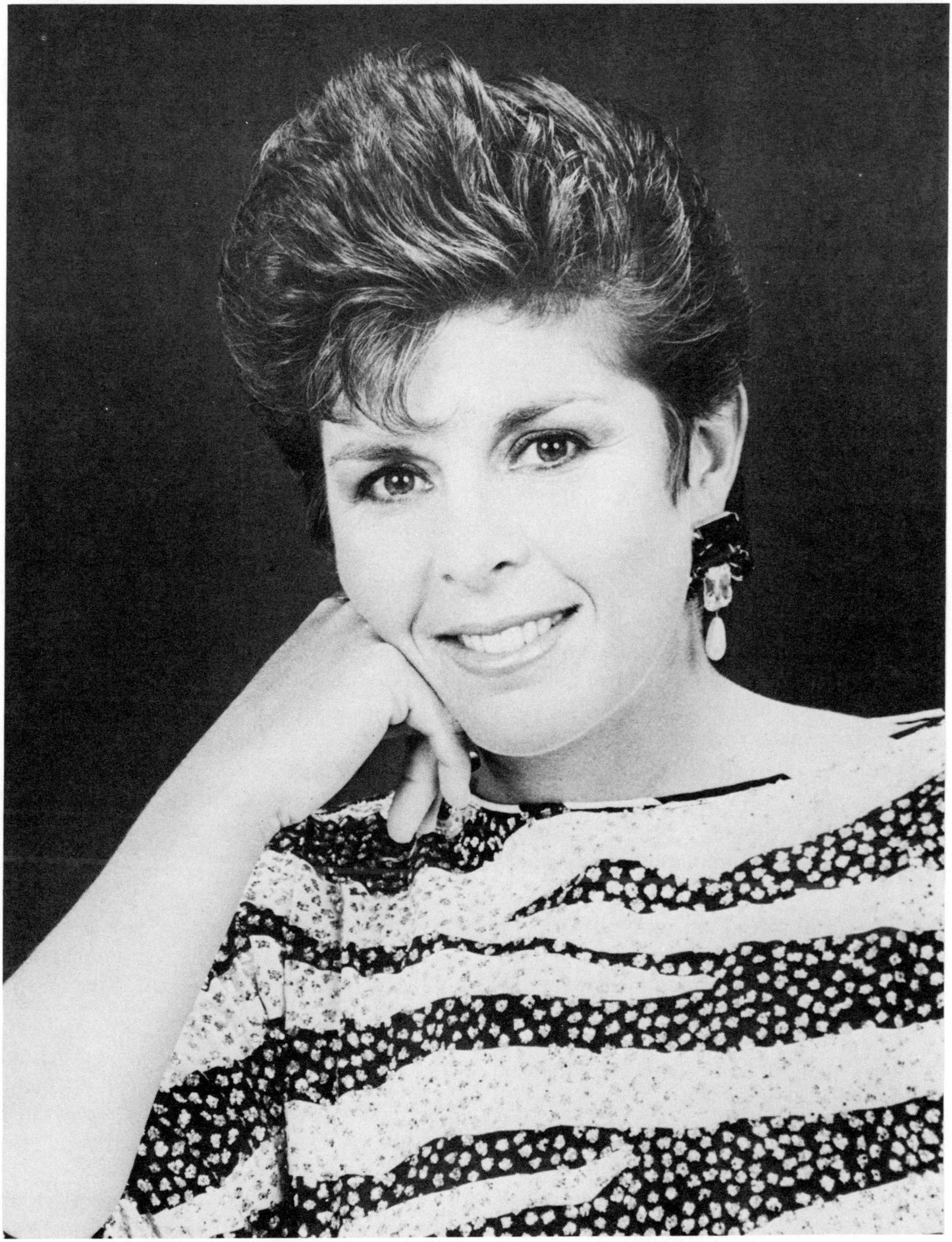

HOLLIS STACY

CANDY COSTIE

HAIR: medium- to finely-textured with a slight wave, highlighted, cut short in layers.

STYLING AIDS: mousse; hair spray; blow-dryer; curling iron.

METHOD:

- Apply mousse to wet hair.
- With head bent forward, blow-dry on high speed, using fingers to push all the nape hair toward the top of the head, for as much volume from the root area as possible (you need lots of volume for this hairstyle).
- While your head is still down, hold the crown section away from scalp, tugging gently and scrunching as you dry your head completely in this position.
- Place your head upright, and apply some hair spray, primarily at the temples. Use your fingers to lift the temple hair up and away from your face (see Chapter 5 for instructions). At the same time, hit that hair with air from your dryer.
- Then, with your fingers, scrunch the rest of the ends all over your head.
- If your hair, like Candy's, has only a slight wave, go over the front section with a curling iron to add more interest and texture.
- Finally, backbrush slightly where you used the curling iron to break up the curls, softening the line, and add another blast or two of hair spray to give the wisps around your face more definition.

  To turn this into a more sophisticated hairstyle, you'll have to use a plastic spray bottle of water, a round styling brush, and a comb.
- Brush all the hair away from your face, using your round brush and blow-dryer to stretch the curl pattern and loosen up the whole line.
- Then give your hair an overall light mist with water, and use your comb to smooth the hair at the temples close to your head, sweeping toward the nape, and to make a side part.

  To get the wave on top, work with the front area in sections:

- Starting closer to the part, wrap a large section of hair around your styling brush, going diagonally back (on an angle away from the part).
- Apply some heat with your blow-dryer on low speed, and gently pull the brush through, stretching the hair into a soft wave.
- Repeat the process with the next section of hair at the front furthest from the part, following the same movements in the same direction, so you wind up with one sweeping, graceful wave.
- Then spray all over lightly with hair spray.

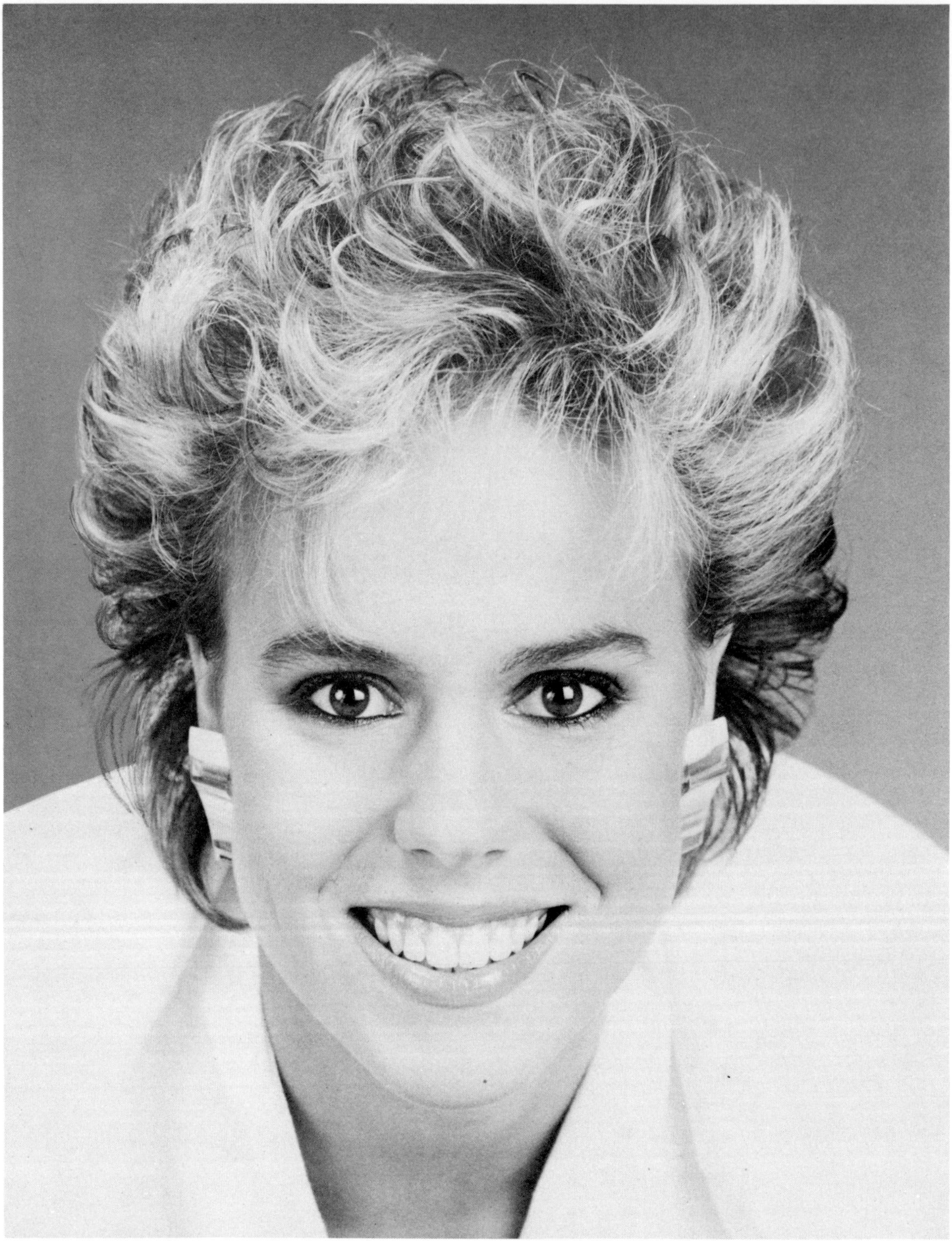

CANDY COSTIE

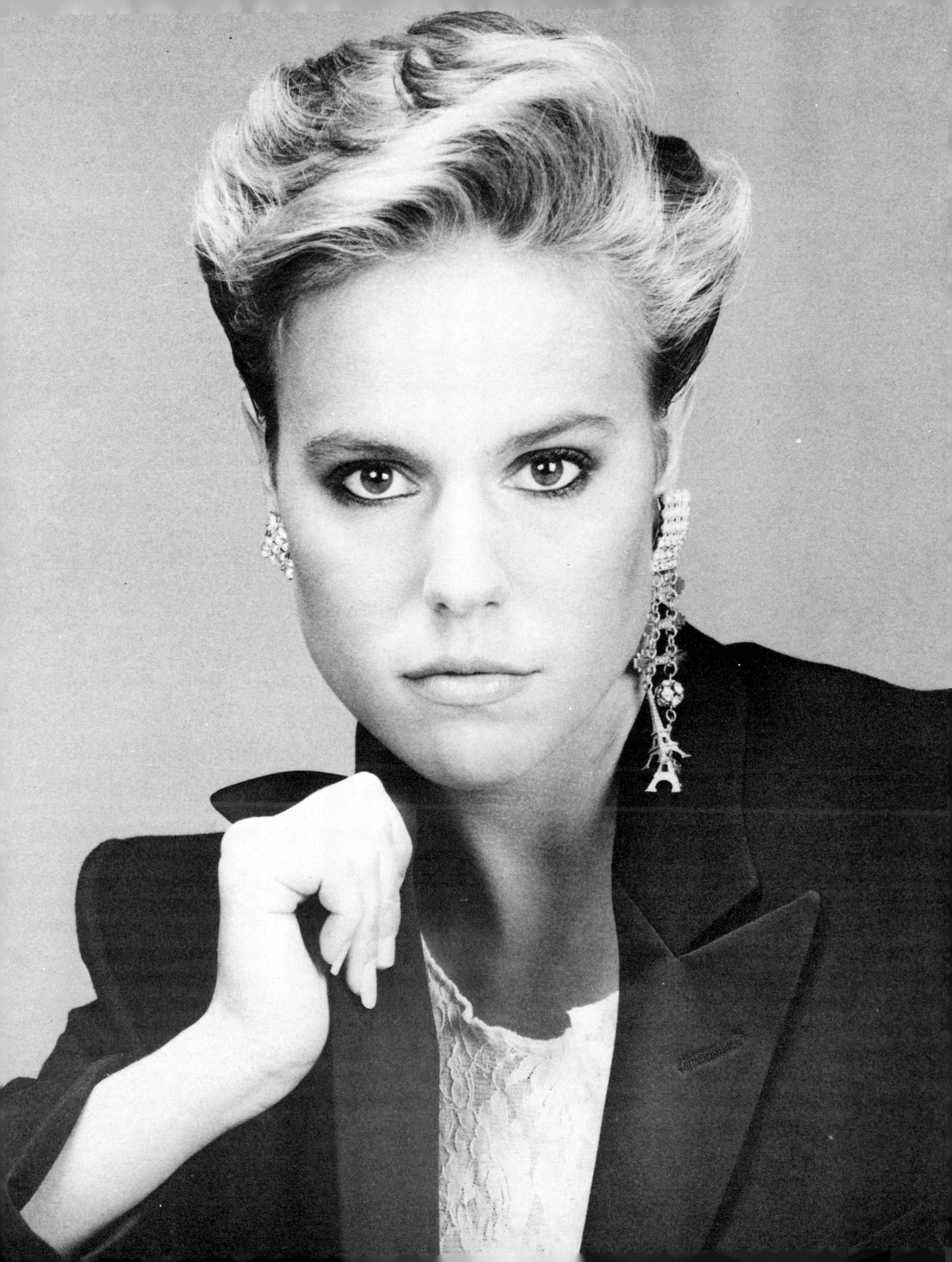

EIGHT

A PERMANENT SOLUTION

If ever a hairstyling subject stirred up strong reactions, it's permanent-waving. In my experience women rarely straddle the fence on this issue. The eager beavers, convinced that a perm will solve all their straight-hair problems, tend to imagine themselves forever blessed with the lush waves or soft curls they've coveted since who knows when. The naysayers, on the other hand, adamantly opposed at the very mention of permanent-waving, can only envision the tight, frizzy little curls made famous by the heroine of film and funnies, Little Orphan Annie.

The truth is, either one or neither one could result. For what you get from a permanent wave—indeed, whether or not you're a good candidate for one—depends entirely on three issues: the kind of hair you have, the kind of hair you want, and the competence of the person perming your hair.

Actually a hairdresser who knows his or her business also knows when *not* to give a perm no matter how much a client wants one. A pretty law student who definitely was *not* a candidate for permanent-waving implored me, for months on end, to perm her superfine, almost transparent titian tresses that fell in one shiny length below her shoulders. I thought with her delicate hair a permanent wave was risky at best. The cortex at the center of each of those silky hair shafts (where the curling action takes place) was so slender that she almost had none. Fearing that the cuticle layer might take the brunt of the waving lotion's effects and would suffer damage, I continually refused. She finally went elsewhere to have it done.

A week or two later she returned with the ends of her hair almost melted away. The rest wasn't in terrific shape either, but we managed to salvage her hair with radical layering, extensive conditioning, and lots of patience on her part until the damaged hair grew out.

Certainly, most hair, including hair on the fine side, doesn't respond that way to chemical treatments administered correctly. But if your hair, like the law student's, leans more toward fragile than fine, or if it's in such poor condition you can't get even a wide-tooth comb through it when it's wet, don't be surprised if your hairstylist advises against perming. *And heed that advice,* especially in summer, when your hair gets lots of sun exposure. After all, wouldn't he or she gladly take your money for that service if it were in your best interests?

For those who can perm their hair, on the other hand, today's permanent wave lotions are far superior to those used as recently as five years ago. Suzy Chaffee and Chris Evert Lloyd are just two examples of active women (with fine hair, in fact) who have enjoyed considerable success with permanent-waving. Suzy now has both the versatility she never had with straight hair and the ease of handling when her set loses its shape after a day's exposure to wet, windy weather on the ski slopes.

"Sometimes it bounces back," she says, "but even when it doesn't, I now can handle my own hair well enough to feel really terrific about how I look."

Permanent-waving for body produces wash-and-wear hair for world champion roller skater April Allen. And her rather straight, medium-textured-hair-turned-wavy requires no fussing whatever unless she *chooses* to fuss. "With a perm I can just let my hair dry naturally while I dress or apply makeup, and it looks terrific," says April. While she loves the look and low maintenance feature of her perm in its "natural" state for every day, April also values the styling flexibility it gives her. "I can always blow it out into smoother styles for dressy occasions," she says. If you find, as these women obviously did, that straight hair isn't your most versatile, easy-care option for an active life-style, a permanent wave could solve your problem in more ways than one.

First, it gives your hair more body and could bring it closer to a middle range in texture and wave pattern. Beyond that, a perm tends to make your hair feel less oily since waving lotions, like hair-coloring agents, lift the hair shaft's cuticle layer, increasing its porosity. And porous hair is drier hair.

Despite the potential benefits, though, before you choose to have a perm, you should know your hair and understand how a permanent wave, or a body wave

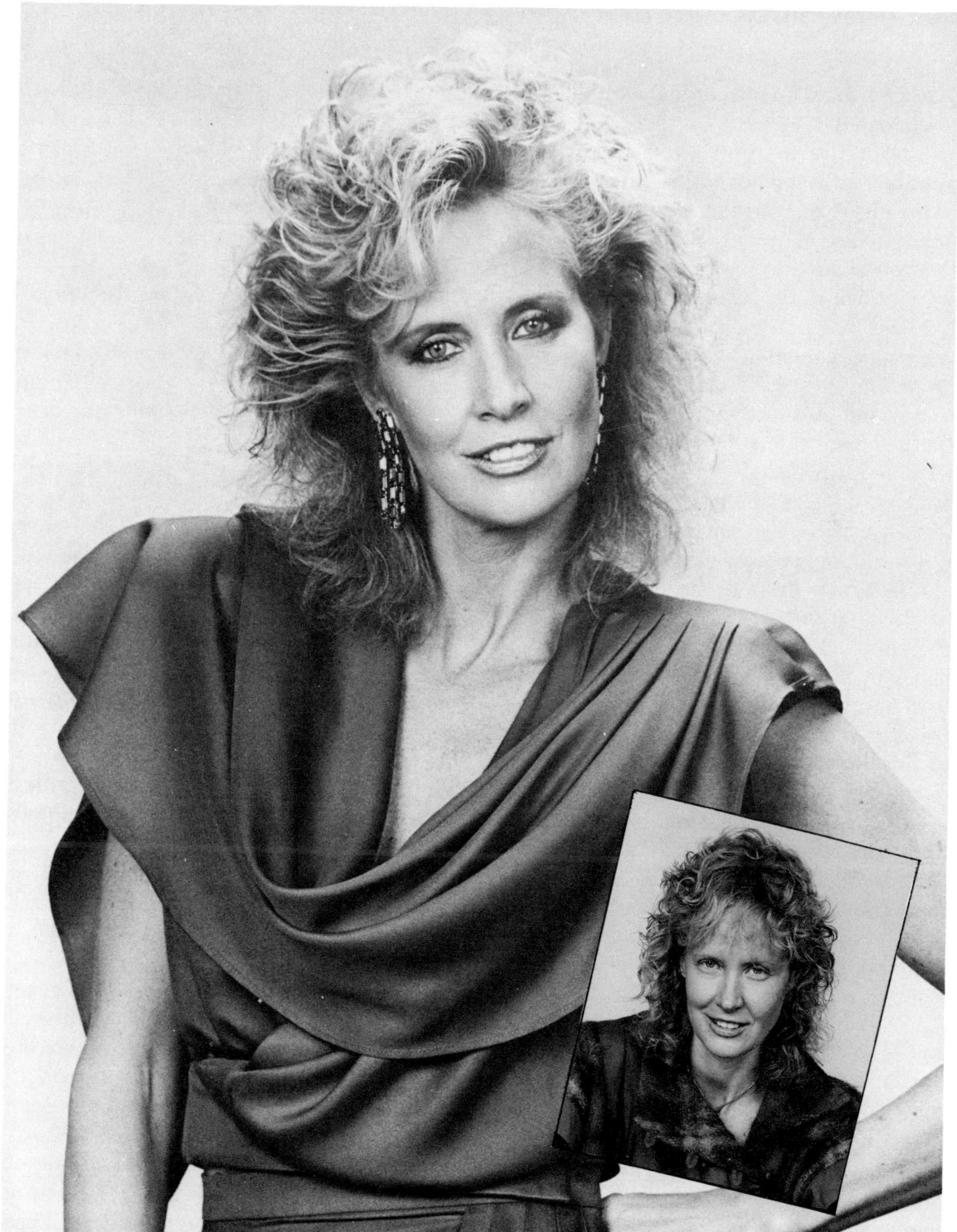

Get a great perm, and even wash-and-wear can work in a pinch. Suzy can easily get by with her perm *au naturel* (see inset), or else, for an evening look she can add a lift here and a scrunch there.

(a perm wound on fatter rods) would work to change it.

Just as water allows you to reshape your hair so that when it dries, it conforms to the shape of the roller you use, permanent-waving solutions induce changes in the hair shaft that permit you to re-form straight hair into a curled pattern. But unlike the temporary change you get with water, permanent-waving solutions rely on strong chemicals that reach into the cortex and alter the structure of the hair shaft more or less permanently. That's why you can disrupt a temporary setting done with water simply by wetting it, but with a perm, your hair has to grow out if you no longer want it.

How curly or loose the perm turns out has little to do with how long you leave the solution on your hair. One person's hair can "take" somewhat more quickly than another's, but thanks to the new superior permanent wave lotions, we're able to fine-tune the whole process, virtually removing the guesswork in timing. Many products today are self-timing, so their action stops automatically after a prescribed period. Beyond this feature, most solutions come in different formulas for virgin hair and for color-treated hair, which, more porous than untreated hair, tends to respond more quickly.

The size of the rods used determines just how curly or wavy a perm will turn out. The smallest permanent wave rods form the tightest curls, whereas the largest rods produce the loose pattern called a body wave. As a student I was taught to wind everything on the tiniest rods. That was okay then because we were perming

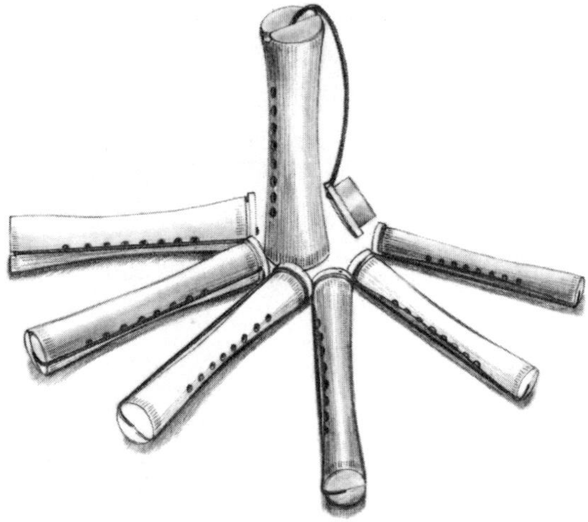

for the frizzy looks that were fashionable years ago.

Perms still enjoy considerable popularity for a different reason. Wound on much larger rods, they can give you great control over hair that once was limp and unmanageable, enhancing its stylability. And although even body wave rods may not seem all that large to you (compared with the fat rollers you're used to seeing), they are proportioned to produce the complete S patterns you need for a proper wave.

Whether you want soft, fluffy curls or a body wave, the success of a perm depends largely on how well the hair is wound on those rods. Unlike ordinary setting on regular rollers, winding for a perm demands considerable skill acquired through training and practice—an excellent reason to have a professional do it.

That doesn't mean you can't get good results with a home permanent kit. Although permanent-waving takes some of the strongest chemicals used for treating hair, home permanents usually contain milder solutions than those formulated for professional use, significantly reducing the risk of hair damage and other mishaps at unskilled hands. Recently a client of mine sailed into the salon with a brand-new home permanent that looked terrific. But before she attempted to use one (with the help of a friend who wound the inaccessible sections at the back of her head), she had asked my advice about the hair she had versus the hair she wanted and what it would take in terms of processing to acquire and maintain it.

So before you pour that permanent wave lotion all over your head—before you attempt *any* home hair treatment with chemicals—get professional advice, read the package directions carefully, and follow them scrupulously.

One feature common to both home and salon permanents: Waving lotions make your hair more susceptible not only to drying but to oxidation, which usually produces unwanted color changes. And frequent exposure to the sun compounds the problem. So whether you perm at home or have a professional do it, pay more attention than ever before to conditioning and other aspects of your hair care program.

Diligent attention to conditioning becomes equally crucial to keeping your hair healthy and manageable if you use chemical hair relaxers to straighten supercurly hair. This process can be highly successful for black women's coarse-textured hair. Leslie Allen, the first black woman to win a major tennis tournament since Althea Gibson's 1958 U.S. Open and Wimbledon victories (the $125,000 Avon purse she snagged in 1981), credits chemical straightening for the handling ease she enjoys and the ability to vary her hairstyle.

"If I left my thick hair in its natural curl, I'd have to keep it very short, limiting me to the one look. With straightening I can wear my hair at a good length for quick-styling options that get me out of the house or the locker room fast," she says, adding that she either can blow it dry straight and wear it up or down or can set it on rollers for curls or waves. "But no matter how I style it, the process is a lot easier and faster than if I were to try to do the same thing with my natural curl."

Despite Leslie's obvious success with this process, with few exceptions, I don't recommend chemical straightening for Caucasians. I have seen very few successful hair-straightening treatments on white women.

Actually, even with an ultracoarse hair texture, if you're active and have to squeeze grooming into a hectic daily schedule, ordinary chemical straightening may not be your most efficient choice. Keeping up with new growth demands regular touch-ups, and the curlier your hair, the more often you have to zap those roots with chemicals to avoid a sharp contrast between the older straightened hair and the newer curly area. So you wind up placing stress on your schedule and your scalp.

Another way to bring your hair closer to the middle-range ideal wave pattern is to relax your kinky hair into a softer look with a curly perm. In this process, for black women, a hair-relaxing agent usually goes

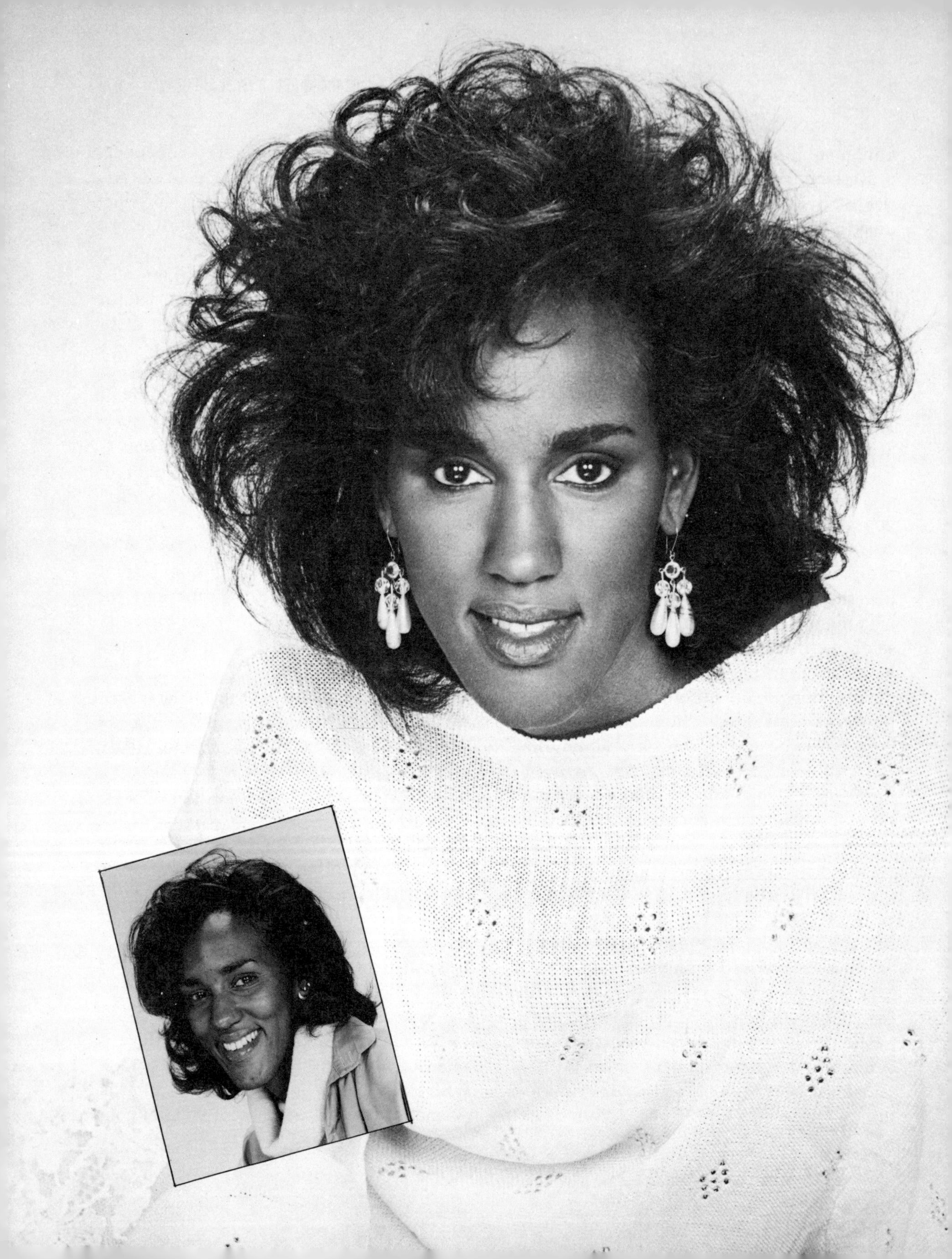

on first (white women with less coarse hair can often skip this step). Then your hairstylist would immediately wind your hair on the largest rods and saturate it with a permanent wave solution to produce a body wave.

The result is a looser, bigger curl that gives you greater styling flexibility with a lot less fuss than you had to invest with kinky hair. Indeed, with a curly perm you can even style your hair for smoothness in specific areas (at the temples and the nape, for example) in less than half the time you would have spent to achieve that look with what nature gave you. And while the curly perm to relax hair usually takes double processing, the results last for four to six months as opposed to the mere six- to eight-week touch-up intervals for standard hair-relaxing techniques.

I favor salon treatments over the do-it-yourself variety in this case as well.

But whether you ultimately choose a salon process or go the home treatment route as a means of making your hair manageable, you'd do well to do some homework in advance. First ask *yourself:*

a. What don't you like about your hair's present behavior (what kind of hair do you have?)?
b. How would you like it to behave instead (what kind of hair do you want?)?

Then consult a qualified professional, and ask *him or her:*

a. Is your goal realistic with your hair type?
b. If not, can you at least reach a happy medium with the help of a perm or a relaxer?
c. Can your hair be permed or relaxed successfully?
d. If so, what kind of process will get the result you want: a perm wound on small rods or a body wave permed on fatter rods, a chemical straightener or the curly perm approach to relaxing?

Answering these questions beforehand can help you avoid dissatisfaction afterward by leading you to the optimum "permanent solution" for your hair management dilemma.

Leslie Allen's chemically straightened hair, shown in its most relaxed state—before styling (see insert), will give her many more hairstyle options than her natural curls would allow.

NINE

REV UP YOUR HAIR COLOR

Few physical improvements can do more for your looks or your outlook than altering the color of your hair. In my experience, even the most reluctant individuals who finally take the plunge after considerable hemming and hawing invariably wonder why they didn't do it ages ago.

The chief reason in most cases is the belief that tinting their hair will make them slaves to it. Some women who use hair color may tell you they *are* slaves to it, but it doesn't have to be that way.

Hair coloring has improved right along with most other segments of the hair care industry; today there is a broader choice of tinting techniques than ever before. Several produce glorious results yet can easily fit into the hectic lives women lead today. The trick is to figure out which one will accomplish both objectives for you.

That boils down to two basic lessons, if you'll be coloring for the first time or you want a better method than the one you've been using: Seek professional advice *first*—especially if you plan to tint your own hair. A colorist can guide you to the correct shade for the results you want. Hair colors shown on packages are based on tints applied to hair stripped virtually white. So what you see on the package isn't the shade you'll get on your present hair color.

Lesson number two: Always opt for a moderate color change rather than a drastic one. Martina Navratilova's golden hair illustrates this point. It works well for her because her natural shade isn't much darker, so her new growth goes almost unnoticed for a considerable time even though she's constantly in the limelight. Consequently Martina can maintain her hair color easily with a single-process touch-up about every four to six weeks. A greater contrast would stand out immediately, demanding attention as often as every three weeks.

Really stark differences between new growth and tinted hair, such as we get with brunettes-turned-blond, create bigger hassles yet. They often require double processing (first lightening, then toning to the desired cast) with every touch-up. This routine can put a crimp into any busy schedule. Drastic color changes that bog you down with such slavish rituals probably aren't for you.

Then why color your hair at all? For the cosmetic benefits obtainable with *subtle* changes. Just as you use makeup to enhance your skin tone, a rich new shade of hair that complements your natural coloring can bring a healthy glow to your face, make your eyes sparkle, or highlight the curve of your cheekbones.

From a strictly practical viewpoint, coloring your hair, believe it or not, can produce certain economic benefits along with a fresh, new look. Studies of physical attractiveness demonstrate that whether it's right or wrong, tinting graying hair can make the difference between landing a job or a promotion and losing out on one—often to a younger-looking individual. On reflection employers interviewed admitted that without any intent to discriminate and with most other qualifications relatively equal, they tended to favor younger-looking job applicants. Several cited gray or graying hair as the most immediately visible factor in what they felt was a largely unconscious response.

Tinting also adds body to your hair because most coloring agents tend to lift your cuticle layers, swelling the hair shafts. That bodybuilding capability provided a substantial beauty bonus for Martina's baby-fine hair.

When I first met her, Martina had a few highlights in her dark blond tresses. We added highlights almost as much to "thicken" her hair as to lighten it. She was so pleased with both effects that she soon lightened all her hair.

You can get eminently pleasing results with hair color, too. And you'll get the ultimate benefit when the way you feel about your lovely new look puts a little more oomph into everything you do. If you don't believe that can happen, just ask professional golfer and past president of the Ladies Professional Golf Association Players' Council Debbie Massey, for whom blond highlights woven subtly into her once mousy, lifeless hair ("which simply didn't mesh with my personality") reinforced her self-image as a doer and achiever. At times during her stint with the association, Massey says, just looking in the mirror renewed her energy, better enabling her to fulfill the double-duty demands of both tournament play and her official position.

"It was exciting and rewarding to see in my reflection someone who *looked* very capable since I filled so much of my time working on my game or on association business," she explains. "Although I felt tired, just looking as if I could do more gave me the impetus I needed to go on, which really made me feel great."

But then the use of hair color changes to improve upon nature and boost one's self-image isn't exactly a new notion. Ever since the first African herdsmen muddied the earth and smeared yellow, orange, and red ocher in their hair—as much, anthropologists say, to identify with a group or to proclaim their position in the hierarchy as to adorn themselves—human beings have sought to alter the color of their tresses. Of course, twentieth-century hair-tinting techniques are vast improvements over those early attempts to embellish hair with pigments. And the social implications of hair color have shifted with time. But not everyone has always viewed the practice favorably.

Thanks to the rather dubious connotation attached to "bleaching" or "dyeing" one's hair in the thirties, relatively few brave souls dared emulate Hollywood's "Blond Bombshell" Jean Harlow. In fact, not until the fifties did such diverse role models as Marilyn Monroe, Doris Day, Arlene Dahl, and Lucille Ball demonstrate that sporting *vivid* hairdos had little to do with wantonness and everything to do with looking and feeling glamorous, wholesome, exotic, sweet, sophisticated, innocent—or just plain beautiful. Following their example, women flocked to "beauty parlors" to turn their tresses anywhere from platinum blond to flaming red even to jet black, inspired by the raven-haired beauty of Elizabeth Taylor.

Toward the middle sixties heads began to turn from Hollywood's glitter to more profound issues raised by peace marchers and naturalist countercultures. Enter the "flower children," bent more on accepting Mother Nature at face value than giving her a helping hand.

Their influence, felt through the seventies, didn't further the industry's growth, but neither did it sound the death knell for artificial hair colors. Granted, relatively few new users joined the women already tinting their hair, who had toned down to more natural-looking shades. Still, by the end of the seventies, punk rockers—their hair aglow in orange, violet, pink, blue, and green—had signaled the start of the pendulum's swing back to hair coloring.

Not that most people want those rainbow hair hues. But the fashion for vibrant hair has reached well beyond the punk rock scene. It didn't take us very long, for example, to grow quite used to the sight of Cyndi Lauper having all that fun (move over, blondes!) in her gaudy getups made all the more so by the splash of blazing colors about her head.

Next to those hues, tinted hair in conventional shades seem innocuous enough. And totally unembellished hair can look downright dull. Both factors have contributed to a rising demand for color-enriched hair that strikes a happy medium

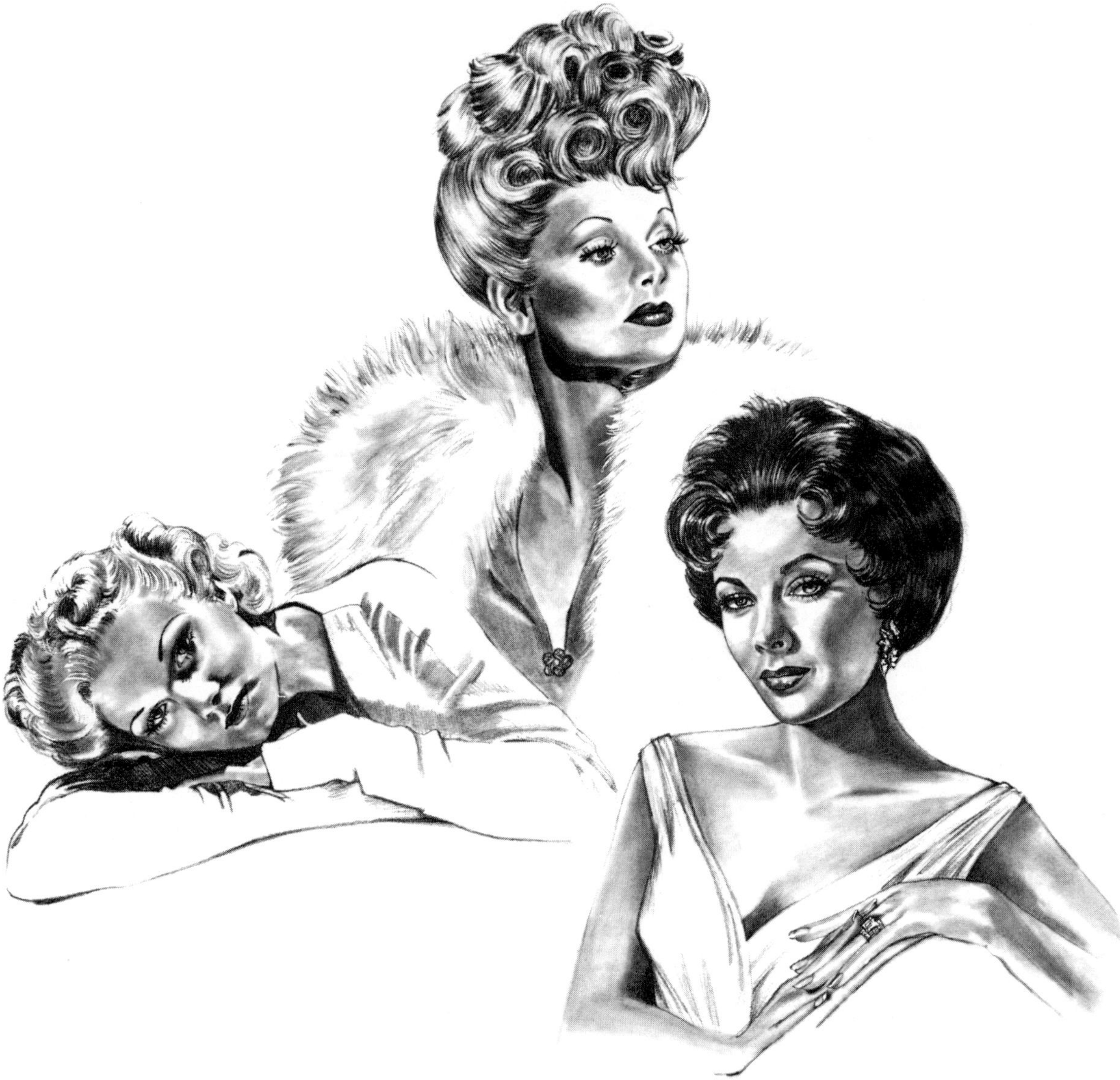

between those bold fifties tones and the pure naturalness of the seventies.

The women most drawn to them are baby boomers. Now in their middle to late thirties, they are fast joining the ranks of the graying.

To be sure, not all the thirty-three million or so women in the United States (and who knows how many worldwide?) who color their hair are turning gray. Some simply desire a change, others want to perk up dull or mousy hair, and still others may be striving for a particular effect—to look more youthful, exotic, sportive or perhaps to emulate an idol.

Whatever your reasons, today you have access to numerous hair-tinting techniques developed for a variety of effects. Whether you color your own hair or have it done professionally, you should get to know the differences and how each product category works. How else can you select the one that will do the most for you with the lowest investment of time and effort?

Temporary color rinses can't even qualify to compete for your attention. They coat your hair with an artificial-looking pigment that lasts only from one shampoo to the next. To maintain their effect, you must repeat the process every time you shampoo—clearly a waste of time especially when you shampoo daily or at least several times a week.

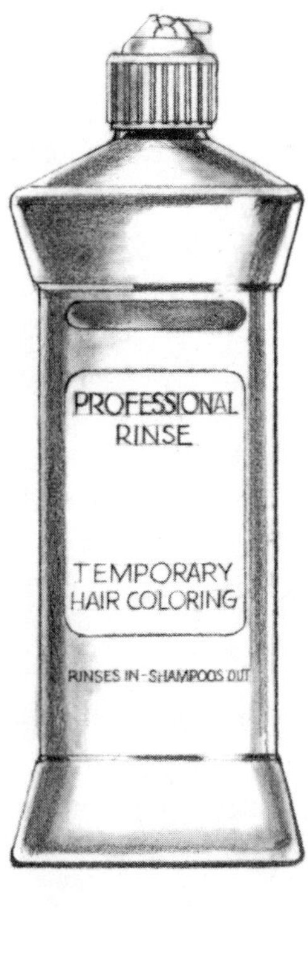

Another drawback: Temporary rinses tend to rub off on your combs and brushes, sometimes on your collars, and most of all, on your pillowcases. So, unless you want to redecorate your bedroom to match your hair, choose a better way to color it.

Semipermanent hair-coloring agents last through four to six shampoos, won't rub off on anything, and provide a more reliable way to rev up your hair color. They're especially good for covering gray if you have twenty-five percent or less gray hair. More than that, in my opinion, calls for a different method, which I'll discuss later on.

Semipermanents come in liquids, foams, and gels squeezed from tubes and are as easy to apply as shampoo. This ease of application can eventually produce color buildup, but that's not an insurmountable problem.

Since they contain no peroxide, semipermanent coloring agents can match your natural shade or darken it—but they never lighten it. So using a light color on dark hair is pointless; it won't show up at all.

Ironically, this aspect of semipermanent tints provides a quick and easy way to put highlights into moderately graying hair. In fact, I used this method when golf pro Dot Germaine decided to cover a small amount of gray in her light brown hair. Only the gray picked up the blond (we chose a color two shades lighter than her

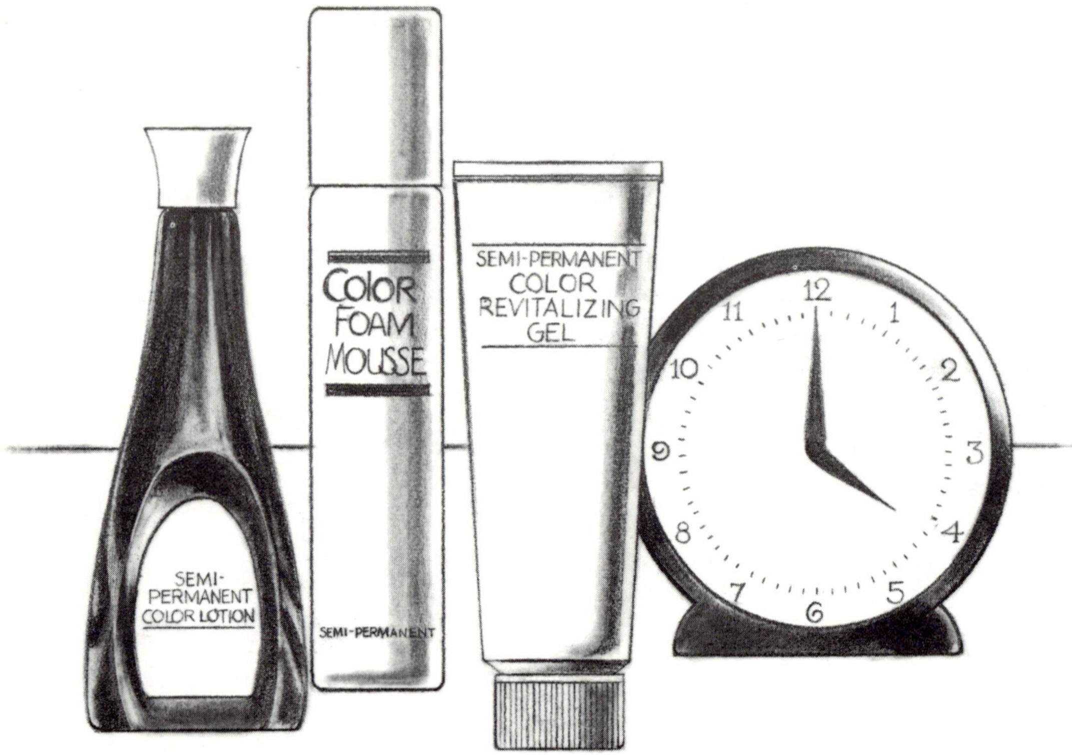

dominant brown) creating just the highlights she wanted.

Henna, a vegetable dye that produces subtler yet longer-lasting results (for up to two months), can achieve a similar effect on sparsely graying hair. It works best on medium to very dark brown shades (with or without a hint of gray), and it doesn't induce an obvious color change. Henna pigments show up against gray yet are barely visible against dark shades (much like bright cellophane wrappers against plain white paper versus dark backgrounds). Hit them with light, however, and you produce lovely, translucent highlights, even against the darkest colors.

Today hennas come in gold and brown tones as well as the familiar red and are great to rev up your natural color without really changing it. I especially like them for hair that gets lots of sun exposure. The pigment coating tends to build up each hair shaft, protecting it and giving fine, weak hair more body. Also, it smooths the cuticle layer, creating a beautiful shine. All are distinct advantages when you're engaged in an activity that has you out in the sun often.

If you choose this route to color enhancing, look for a hundred percent natural or organic henna, which will need an outside heat source to develop. (The ancient Egyptians let the sun bake it in, but

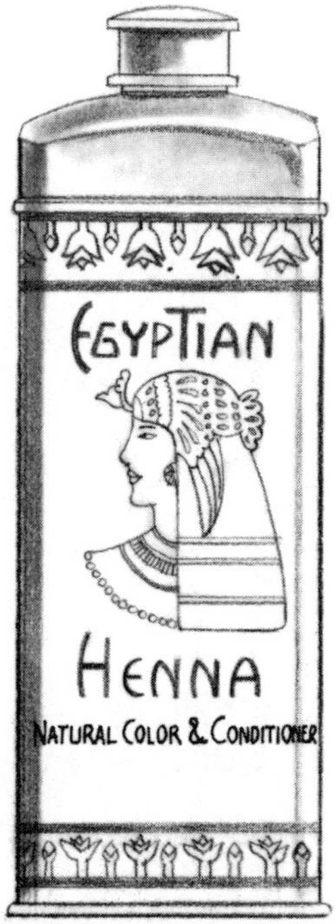

your hair dryer will do just fine.) So, if the package directions boast "No need to sit under a dryer" or something similar, the product contains an activating chemical and isn't all natural.

Single-process permanent tints come in liquid and in easier-to-apply shampoo-in formulas. I favor this product category for most color changes—including tinting gray hair—for several reasons:

First, these formulas are peroxide-based, so you can use them not only to darken your color or to rev it up but to lighten it a shade or two. Any more than that would need double processing (lightening, then toning) and would show your roots too often.

Another advantage is that permanent tints don't wash out. So you reapply only when new growth becomes obvious. And unless you shampoo in your color, *you retouch only the roots for the full developing period.* You pull the color through the rest of your hair briefly, just to freshen it. Since *subtle* color changes tend to camouflage your roots, they could allow you as many as six to eight weeks, sometimes longer, between touch-ups.

Substantially gray roots, however, may show up enough against tinted areas to demand retouching every three to four weeks (hair grows about a half inch a month). So, with more than twenty-five percent gray, your hair will blend best with lighter tints, regardless of your original natural color.

Whatever shade you use, permanent tints are your most viable approach to covering that much gray since they don't wash out. With a product that does, the gray throughout your hair would reappear constantly as the color fades.

Yet another benefit of permanent haircoloring agents is that they produce more natural-looking tones. Because you retouch primarily the roots, you don't get color buildup. This problem occurs when layers of color accumulate at the ends of the hair with repeated applications of any shampoo-in hair-coloring agent, whether it's semipermanent or permanent. The result is a muddy, uneven color that can start to show up after the third or fourth application.

Although semipermanent colors last through only six or so shampoos, they don't wash out completely. And permanent tints don't wash out at all. So in slath-

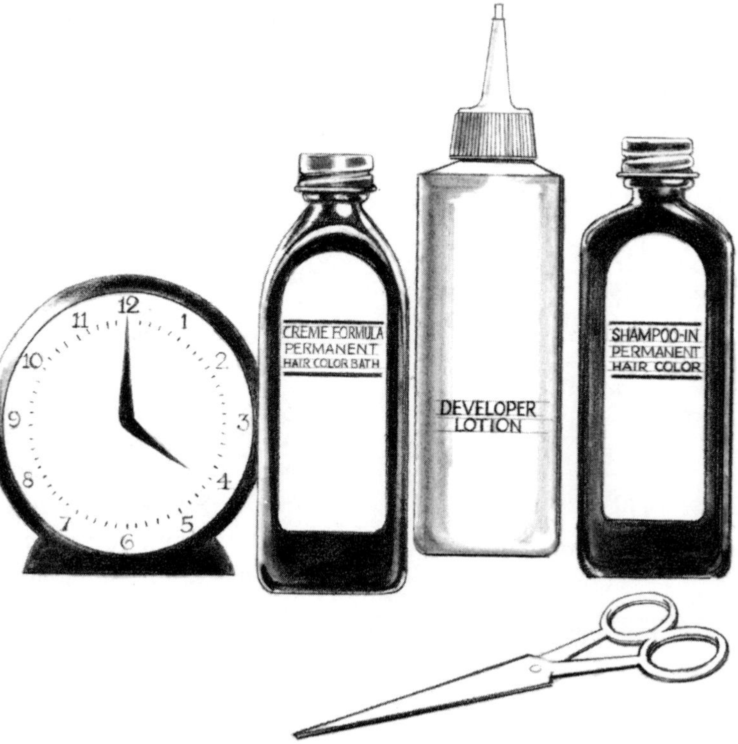

ering your entire head of hair every time you color it, you apply new tint on top of the old. In addition, your color-treated hair, always more porous than virgin hair, grabs the new application much faster than your roots do. So the color gets too much developing time, further intensifying the shade at the ends.

Overtreating too porous hair can lead to much bigger problems, as I learned when I was still in training and inexperienced. Valerie, a six-foot-tall and very slender model I used in Florida, had ultra-pale skin. She also had black hair, which I colored strawberry blond, a favorite shade for competition models. Between competitive events we retouched her hair as often as every other week, but during the events we spruced up her color twice within a single week. Her hair was overtreated, to say the least. But neither of us realized *how* overtreated until the awful day she was booked for a Burdine's promotion at which the models were to portray mannequins.

At her normal touch-up, just hours before the booking, we decided to brighten her shade a bit. I pulled the color right to the ends of her hair and left it there for almost the entire developing time.

Upon rinsing it out, I gaped in horror. Her root hair was the strawberry blond we wanted, but the ends were so porous they had grabbed only the base pigment (the primary color component in most hair-coloring agents). They had turned *purple.*

Wacky hair colors weren't a fad then as they are these days. So the effect of that purple hair, rimmed in strawberry blonde, against her porcelain complexion was frightening. And to say it upset Valerie understates her tearful reaction—especially when she realized that any attempt to correct the color of that still highly porous hair would produce the same result or worse. Besides, she was expected at Burdine's in less than an hour.

What to do? The only thing I could do just then: I created a breathtaking style for her avant-garde hair and drove a still-fretting Valerie to her booking.

The people in charge at Burdine's believed we had improvised the grotesque look especially for her stint as a mannequin, which earned Valerie praise for initiative. And I suppose you could say she also impressed the poor, unsuspecting customers: They almost passed out when the six-foot-tall, skinny "mannequin" done up with chalky skin and purple-to-strawberry blond hair suddenly smiled and winked at them.

That is not to say that in coloring porous hair, you're likely to shock your friends by turning it purple or green, although if you abuse your hair enough, it could happen. Valerie's sad tale reiterates an important lesson: Seek professional guidance from an experienced colorist before you attempt to use any hair-coloring agent.

For the most reliable advice, be sure to spell out your recent hair care history (perms, hair coloring, and so on) as well as any health condition or medication you think might affect the outcome. If you tint at home, don't ignore package directives for skin patch tests or hair strand tests no matter how many times you've used the particular product before. The formula, your hair, your chemistry, or all three could have changed enough to alter your result or produce a reaction you didn't have before.

Of course, color buildup, by far the most common dilemma with porous hair, is a petty annoyance compared to Valerie's disaster. Chances are you can shampoo in color two or three, even four times before it begins to show. But beyond that I recommend applying it as you would a standard liquid formula, which many women use quite successfully at home. In other words, color the roots, and only after the appropriate developing time, work the product through the rest of your hair just long enough to freshen the shade.

Admittedly the sectioning and parting this procedure requires take more time and more effort if you do your own hair. But that's another reason to opt for the most subtle hair color changes and to use the longest-lasting coloring agents. And even if you do color at home, why do it all yourself? I know several women whose husbands help out with the hard-to-reach areas at the back of their heads. One regularly enlists the aid of her teenage daughter. Still another trades off with a friend.

You can use the buddy system, too. Find a partner who also colors her hair.

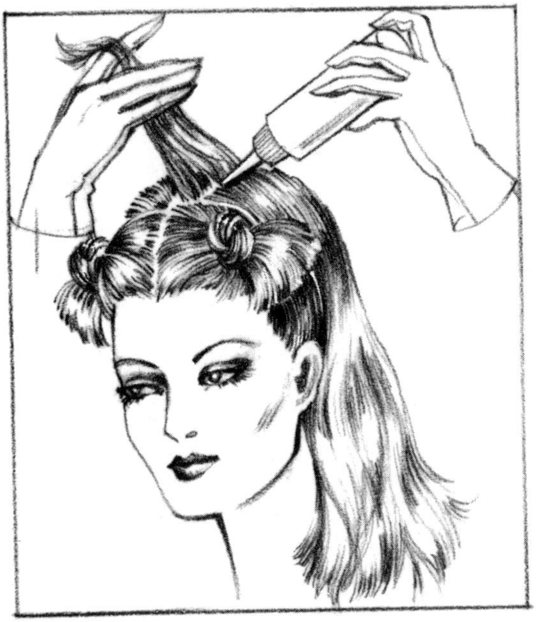

Do it together, and help each other out. You'll both save time and wind up with better results.

Highlighting, the permanent hair-coloring technique that has my heartiest recommendation, especially for an active lifestyle, could give you the most satisfying result: a glamorous look that needs minimum upkeep. This procedure—also called streaking, tipping, frosting, naturalizing, or selective shading—involves isolating strands of hair and lifting them several shades lighter than your natural color. To be truly effective, highlighting must be gradual. This could be the single most important element to keep in mind if you plan to go this route.

First let's examine why you should. Nature's own brand of highlighting—almost inevitable if you're into tennis, golf, running, swimming, skiing, skating, or any activity that exposes you to lots of sun—would blend successfully with a few well-placed highlights of your own.

But even if you are stuck in a dimly lit office all day, highlighting done well can last months without needing a touch-up simply because new growth tends to blend right in with the overall effect of shading. So you can save not only time but wear and tear on your hair, which already endures sweating, shampooing, blow-drying, and many other stresses with great regularity.

From a purely cosmetic stance, highlighted hair will present you at your very best. To make a distinctive statement, your appearance should reflect your tastes and your interests, which include the things you like to do. What could better enhance your image as a vigorous, active woman

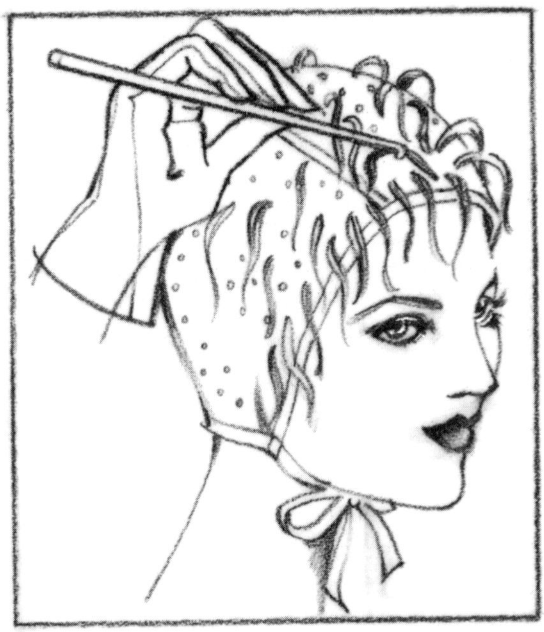

than the attractive, healthy glow that comes with the look of sun-kissed hair?

To achieve that look in the most flattering way possible, you must exercise patience, especially if you do it yourself. And you can—quite successfully—with one of several home highlighting kits on the market.

While this advice may seem to contradict my quick and easy hair care philosophy, it actually underscores it. Your patience at the outset will reward you with an eminently pleasing result that needs very little maintenance. So don't expect to get all your beautiful, subtle blond highlights in one sitting. Starting with all-one-color hair, you could need as many as three or four sessions with a kit to arrive at your desired effect. And it *should* take at least two.

- Start with the strands around your face, at the hairline and up toward the crown area, where the sun would lighten it naturally. Begin by using your lightener about ten or twelve minutes to lift the color just a shade or two on selected strands. A few wisps (only three or four hairs pulled through each hole if you use a cap) are more than adequate at any one sitting.
- Then work gradually toward the back, keeping in mind that ultimately you want a modulation of color—the lightest around your face and at the crown, getting progressively darker toward the back of your head.
- The second time you highlight, you'll build on what you already have by picking up some strands (again no more than three or four hairs) in your natural shade and some that have already been lifted for ten minutes.
- The third time you'll work with some more of your natural hair color as well as strands that were treated for ten minutes in the second session and a few you treated in both previous sessions.

That's how you highlight *gradually,* working up to the effect you want rather than just smearing it on here and there. The darker your hair, the more slowly you should build up to your goal, adding a bit more strategic shading each time you highlight and following package recommendations for intervals between use. The most dramatic effects ultimately will range from your natural color at one end of the spectrum to varying tones in the middle to the palest shade you want at the other end of the spectrum.

How pale should that be? That depends on your natural hair color. You can lift selected strands anywhere from one to, say, eight shades lighter. The longer you leave the lightener on your hair, the paler it will get.

With medium to dark brown hair, for example, you should use a shorter developing time because you want subtler effects. By controlling the process with timing—perhaps leaving the lightener on for only three or four minutes—you could wind up with deep golden highlights, with auburn tones, or with very light browns. Your results will depend on your hair's natural pigment.

Really pale blond highlights will contrast too sharply with a dark color, producing unsightly streaks—a kind of zebra striping that some women liked in the sixties.

A professional colorist has the experience, creative know-how, and wherewithal to balance these light to dark effects successfully in much less time—even a single sitting—than you can manage at home. But whoever highlights your hair, once you get your desired result, maintenance becomes a breeze. Blending new highlights with old ones, much easier than starting from scratch even for do-it-yourselfers, gets simpler with practice.

Whatever hair color you start with, bear in mind that the sun will continue to bleach it to some extent. Resist the temptation to overhighlight so you don't create a flashy look when you want understated elegance.

A "less is more" philosophy will serve you best no matter what hair-coloring technique you use. If you adhere to that axiom and observe the other dos and don'ts of hair tinting set forth in this chapter, more than likely you'll wind up with glorious, color-enriched hair that needs little maintenance and throws a whole new light on your looks—maybe on your life.

TEN

SAVE YOUR OWN SKIN

No matter how you choose to unwind after toiling all week at a desk, behind a counter, or in your own kitchen, more than likely you've joined the hordes who, over the past three or four decades, have been spending much of their leisure time out in the sunshine and fresh air. And whether you hike and climb mountains weekends or lean toward the simpler pleasures in backyard barbecues and Sundays in the park with the kids, all that exposure to the outdoors can affect your skin just as it does your hair. The nature and extent of its impact, of course, depend largely on how well you treat your skin.

With the right care, a face that reflects something of an outdoors life-style can exude a "golden girl" quality (by no means restricted to blondes). Robust color in your cheeks hints at a healthy way of life. You can get this look despite the weekday pallor that descends on most Monday-through-Friday shut-ins.

On the other hand, if you neglect your skin, such a face might show the wear and tear wrought by nature's elements, which can be every bit as unkind to your skin as to your hair, especially after steady doses of drying artificially heated or cooled indoor air. That nastiness can erupt in highly visible blemishes, dry patches, or the lines and wrinkles that betray prematurely aging skin.

I became acutely aware of this destructive potential shortly after I had begun to style hair in Florida, when I discovered that many of my clients were ten years younger than they appeared. As I got to know these women better, I realized my misconceptions had a lot less to do with poor judgment on my part than with their favorite pastimes. Almost without exception, they doggedly followed the sun year-round to indulge their passions for tennis, golf, or just stretching out to soak up those rays. And with their choice of recreation came both the pleasures and the pitfalls of an outdoors life-style.

Certainly my cosmetology training had stressed as much about the threats of sun, wind, and so forth to skin as to hair. But it never quite prepared me for so many vivid examples of what happens when the elements rob our skin—especially faces, hands, and necks—of the moisture it needs to remain soft, smooth, and supple.

Until then, like most people, I had regarded the dermatologists' warnings as overreactive. Now as a beauty professional with considerable hands-on experience, I'm convinced—and I fervently hope to convince you, too—that's not the case. If you engage in activities that keep you outdoors a lot, elements that deplete your hair of moisture pose a similar threat to your skin—sometimes with far more lasting consequences.

Sun exposure, the worst offender by far, can produce skin damage you can't reverse as readily as you can snip off the damaged ends of your hair. Dermatologists blame ultraviolet rays more than any other culprit for the excessive dryness that prematurely etches lines and wrinkles on your face and neck and for other early skin changes we normally associate with aging. Most changes show up on exposed areas, as does skin cancer, another risk to those who love the outdoors, particularly after many years of sporting under the sun.

Although skin cancer is rare among black women, black skin isn't impervious to the sun's drying and aging effects. On the contrary, *all* skin tones, light or dark, will eventually succumb to the aftermath of a steady diet of sunshine: itching, flaking, and unsightly blotching, not to mention sunburn. Obviously the darker your skin, the longer it will tolerate exposure to the sun without burning. But once sunburn occurs, it can be just as raw and painful on dark skin as on light, beginning, as it often does, at the top of your head.

Indeed, whether you spend your summers on horseback or roller skates, the extension of your facial skin called your scalp gets zapped from time to time—especially where your hair parts. So the annoying itch and flaky white stuff you may attribute to a case of dandruff may really be the aftermath of a sunburn.

The risks associated with sun are by no means restricted to warm weather. If the snow season brings out your energetic best, beware the cold white sunlight of winter bouncing up at you from the ski slopes, from a toboggan run, or from the snowman you have built on your front lawn. It can do as much harm as sun reflected off sand and water. In fact, cold-weather rays may be more intense if you pursue winter activities, as many people do, at high altitudes, where the atmosphere is thinner, the air less polluted, and the sun a lot less filtered.

If those cold winter winds send you south instead, you risk sunburn and drying skin not only in desert climates but in the hot, humid tropics or semitropics. Ironically, steps you take to protect your skin from sun, in either setting, can cause other problems. If you slather yourself with a thick coat of oily suntan lotion, then perspire profusely, as is inevitable if you move around in oppressive climates, the oil and your perspiration will mingle and may clog your pores and sweat glands. A common result is the itchy redness of prickly heat.

But excessive drying—water loss from your skin's outer layer and inadequate water replacement from its lower layers—ranks number one among your potential beauty perils.

Abrasive winds on a boat, beach, or mountaintop can give you the rough red skin we call windburn. And if you don't think those balmy breezes can deplete moisture, just ask your grandmother if she didn't like windy days for line-drying laundry fast before we had clothes dryers.

Cold, dry climates you encounter skiing, sledding, or ice-skating also rob your skin of moisture quickly, producing the brittleness and cracking of chapped skin. Hands and face rubbed with snow during accidental tumbles are even more susceptible because wet skin chaps faster.

Frequent showers, another moisture-depleting obstacle to smooth, supple skin, pose a problem because along with dirt and perspiration, all that soap and water tend to wash away our skin's natural moisturizing agents.

Excessively oily skin presents a different sort of dilemma if you perspire profusely. Your perspiration mingles with surface oils, which then tend to spread, making your skin seem even oilier. Indoor activities, such as a game of squash or a strenuous workout, can compound your problem because you don't experience the drying and evaporating effects of the outdoors.

Must you put up with any of these obstacles to gorgeous, glowing skin? I should say not. You can make the two quite compatible with the simplest protective, preventive, and corrective measures.

I see no more magic in maintaining terrific-looking skin under most circumstances than I do in keeping your hair healthy and manageable. Nor do I see a need for elaborate beauty treatments that can consume just as much time as radical hairstyle or hair color changes. And frequent drying showers, for example, may be all it takes to handle an oily skin problem.

I know many active women with gorgeous skin who do little more than cleanse and moisturize. But they do it religiously—before and after playing hard and sometimes during a break, when they replenish moisturizing sunscreen lotions.

Certainly, problem skin needs the attention of a dermatologist. But in most cases a good, basic skin care routine, which shouldn't take more than minutes out of your day, and a few commonsense precautions should give you the optimum natural resource with which to create the fabulous face designs you want quickly and easily. For just as hair in top form will allow you the best styling control, only when your skin is in top condition can you deftly apply those wonderful looks with makeup. After all, you can't work fast and get a terrific result if first you have to busy yourself camouflaging a host of preventable, or at least controllable, flaws in your complexion—those that *can* be hidden, that is.

Of course, the only way to begin is with scrupulously clean skin. But *cleansing your face and neck* is not just a matter of soaping up and rinsing off. Soap-and-water washing depletes your skin's natural oils. So unless you have very oily skin, opt for cleansing creams or lotions for those areas, and then freshen your skin with a *non*alcohol skin toner after you have removed all the cleanser. Faces and necks are vulnerable enough to drying without any extra help from soaps or highly astringent lotions.

Like shampoos, modern cleansing creams and lotions contain different proportions of oil, water, and other ingredients to modify their consistency, texture, and effect on skin. Those formulated for dry skin include components to limit their oil-removing properties; products for oilier skin are made to remove more of your oil secretions.

Superoily skin may need extra help from an astringent toner after cleansing with a cream or from occasional soap-and-water washing—far more effective than cleansing creams at removing oil. I'd recommend you choose a facial soap that can be readily rinsed off, such as a transparent glycerin-based bar.

If you have an oily scalp, more than likely your forehead, nose, and chin (the infamous "T zone") also have overly active oil glands, although the rest of your face may lean toward the dry side. Cleanse your combination skin first and foremost to remove the excess oils. You can lubricate the dry areas afterward with an appropriate moisturizing agent.

Facial cleansers range from heavy cold creams to lighter "cleansing creams," which have less drag on the skin, to the lightest milky lotions and aerosol foams, best for cleansing oily skin. Some even rinse away with water.

No single approach to facial cleansing is the best way. Like shampoos, the cleanser you use is largely a subjective issue. In this instance it depends on how dry or oily your skin feels and the product consistency you prefer.

Your body cleansing routine to minimize dry skin should call not for fewer showers but for faster ones with warm, not hot, water. The hotter the water, the more drying it is. And be sure to rinse thoroughly to remove all traces of soap. Even a slight residue will rob your skin of its oils. If hard water poses a problem in your area, you may find that synthetic detergents such as those found in some body shampoos rinse away more readily.

Moisturizing, the other major component of your antidrying skin care routine, can be somewhat misleading. The creams and lotions you use for this purpose don't actually put moisture into your skin. Only water can truly moisturize. Dermatologists point out that experiments with sections of dry, brittle skin tissue have demonstrated the difference. Even prolonged contact with certain ingredients such as lanolin, commonly found in commercial skin moisturizers, did nothing to restore the tissue's pliability, whereas immersing it in water and exposing the tissue for a time to humid air did.

The next obvious question: How can I say that showers dry the skin when the evidence shows that only water can moisturize it? It's simple. Showers wash away the natural oils that act as a sealant to help skin *retain* moisture from within.

That's where moisturizing agents come in. Like hair conditioners, skin moisturizers pinch-hit for nature's protective coating when your activities deplete it. Therefore, you should never, ever go without the protection of moisturizers on your body and on your face—above all, around the eyes. That part of your face has no oil glands and needs all the help it can get from a good eye cream. Petroleum jelly makes a great one for overnight use, though you might choose a less greasy one for daytime.

Although moisturizers are generally less oily than most cleansing creams, they do contain oil in various amounts, creating an occlusive seal that helps retain some of the replacement moisture from within.

The more oil a product contains, the more effectively it keeps moisture in—or out. So those that contain less oil make a better choice for humid days. They rely more on softening ingredients that help draw water from the air to your skin. Low-humidity days call for a somewhat oilier product. There's little moisture to be pulled from the air on dry days, and you need the extra oil to help you keep what moisture you have.

Here again, the marketplace offers hundreds of products. If you swim, surf, or water-ski a lot, a moisturizer labeled for "extra-dry skin" (which means it contains more oil) probably would make the best stand-in for your skin's natural oils, considering the combined effects of water, sun, and wind. Also, a thin coat of bath oil applied while your skin is still damp from your shower could offer the utmost protection.

Of course, no skin care aid counts more than that which shields your skin from the sun's harmful rays. No one appreciates more than I do the psychological lift to be had from the radiance that accompanies a suntan. But believe me, with the amount of suntime you rack up during ordinary outdoors activities, you can't avoid getting color no matter what you do, short of dressing for a space walk. The only question is how much color you'll get. That depends on the efficiency of your sun-blocking agent and your natural skin pigmentation.

Don't be cavalier about the kind of skin that tans easily. In fact, you'd do very well to shun those deep, muddy skin tones, which tend to take on a purple cast on some black skins. Before you know it, they'll have you looking like parched leather from head to toe. Strive, instead, for the radiant, healthy glow of a complexion barely kissed by the sun. Whether your skin absorbs those rays in minutes or you must build up to a tan gradually, you need supersunscreening help to get and maintain that look.

Today sunblocking preparations contain moisturizing agents and chemical sunscreens not only to slash your sunburn risk but also to reduce the tanning potential that ages skin. They offer different levels of protection, and you can be sure that a product labeled as a tan "promoter" lets through more of the rays than you should want.

None of them is a hundred percent effective, so even a lotion that boasts a maximum protection value of 15 lets through some of the tanning rays. But it also protects your skin from the harmful ultraviolets fifteen times longer than no sunscreen at all. Now you can even get sunscreens specially formulated for hair and scalp.

If you insist on tanning your body darker, use a sunscreen with a protection value no lower than 8. And under all circumstances give your face and neck the highest level of protection available. At this writing, sunblockers, created specifically to handle the outdoor athlete's greatest vulnerabilities, have begun to offer protection as high as 20 for faces and 25 for noses, ears, and lips. You can always blend your body and face with a bronzer or tinted moisturizer and then make it come absolutely alive with a blusher. You'll get a beautiful, healthy glow without changing your skin one iota.

In fact, I see tinted moisturizers as the makeup base of choice over other foundations for true "sports beauty" with or without a tan. They come in light, medium, and dark tones, and you can control the intensity of your chosen shade by the amount you apply. Best of all, they're sheer, light, and natural-looking.

Some women do feel more secure with the sort of "second-skin" coverage they get from opaque foundations, which can provide extra protection against windburn, chapping, and perhaps some shielding from the sun when they contain sunscreens. But unless you choose just the right one for your skin, then use it over a compatible moisturizer, and develop the skills to apply it for the most "dewy" effect, an opaque foundation may seem more artificial than natural, especially under glaring sunlight—not exactly the look you want on a hiking trail or a bike path in the park. Nor are you likely to save time applying or removing it.

My "sports beauty" philosophy embraces a naturalness and simplicity meant to project the best of who you are and to help you do so without cramming your already hectic schedule. You need relatively little equipment to implement it.

I've already discussed cleansing products, moisturizers, and skin toners. Since your face design will be only as fabulous as the skin that shines through it, ignoring these skin care aids will severely handicap you, just as their judicious use will give you an incredible head start. If you haven't been following a good skin care regimen, start now and give your complexion a chance to respond to your tender loving care. With diligent attention, especially before bedtime, within a week or two you'll begin to see wonderful results.

Then, even with one foot constantly

out the door, you'll be able to maintain the looks you love with only the following aids:

- *A cover-up stick or cream* to conceal your imperfections (we all know that no one has flawless skin). The tiniest spec of concealer will spread a very long way; use too much, and you'll have to conceal your concealer. I recommend a cover-up to blend with your finished face design, especially if you're also blending your face with a tanned body. Then you can use it if you need it for quick touch-ups later.
- *A tube of tinted moisturizer* to complement your natural skin tone or to bring your face up to a shade slightly lighter than your tanned body. Anything deeper will look unreal and will fight with your blusher for attention.
- *A translucent, colorless pressed-powder compact* and a small soft but full brush (or a puff) to apply it. You need only the slightest fluff of powder on your nose, forehead and chin to "set" your makeup and reduce shine. Don't powder around your eyes and mouth. Powder tends to collect in even tiny lines and wrinkles, emphasizing them.
- *A powder blusher compact* with a soft, full brush for application. (A creamy lipstick applied with your fingertips can stand in for cheek color in an emergency.)
- *Lip color in a stick or a wand and a tiny pot or stick of colorless or lightly tinted lip gloss* to be used together or separately, depending on the time of day and the effect you want.
- *Two or three tones of eye shadow in a single compact unit* with its own applicator brush or sponge. Choose a subtle color (muted mauve shades rather than bright purples) that you can play down or intensify, depending on the time of day and the occasion.
- *A soft eye pencil in brown* works for almost any skin tone or eye color and always should be your preferred daytime shade. This pencil will do double duty as an eyeliner for daytime and as your eyebrow filler for any time if you need one.
- *A soft eye pencil in black,* which also enhances almost any skin tone or eye color when used for the knockout "sooty" evening effects you want to get with your eyeliner.

Actually, both eye pencils give you lots of flexibility. In a pinch, either one can be blended out over your eyelids for subtle shadow and then used more intensely to line the eyes. And if you choose a dual-color pencil (such as brown on one side with plum on the other or black with pale mauve), you'll get yet more versatility, with no further investment of time.

Some black women I know can do a lot more than white women with colors in place of black or brown for eye shadows and pencils because they can get dramatic yet wonderfully subtle effects with color on their dark complexions. But even in these instances I prefer shades like plum, navy, and muted mauves over bright, harsh colors.

- *A wand of black mascara,* the only color you need for maximum definition, to be applied sparingly for days and more liberally at night. Anything lighter will make little or no impact unless you have the palest skin and eyes.
  I recommend regular mascara simply because it's a lot easier to remove than the waterproof variety. However, if you swim or perspire heavily during sports, a waterproof mascara may be your best option for those activities.
- *A light liquid foundation* to match your skin tone and a sponge to apply it for the velvet-smooth look that will turn your beautiful daytime face into a breathtaking vision for special evenings.

With this relatively modest store of implements you can create and maintain the loveliest looks no matter where you go or how much in a hurry you are to get there. So you can see how my quick and easy concept works, let's look briefly at one of many hectic days in the life of

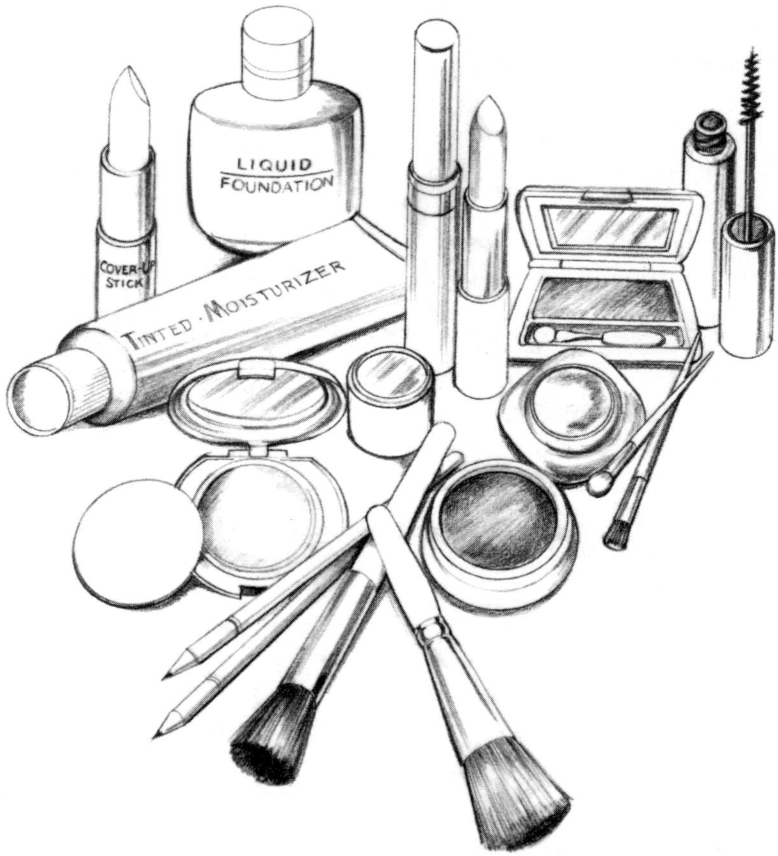

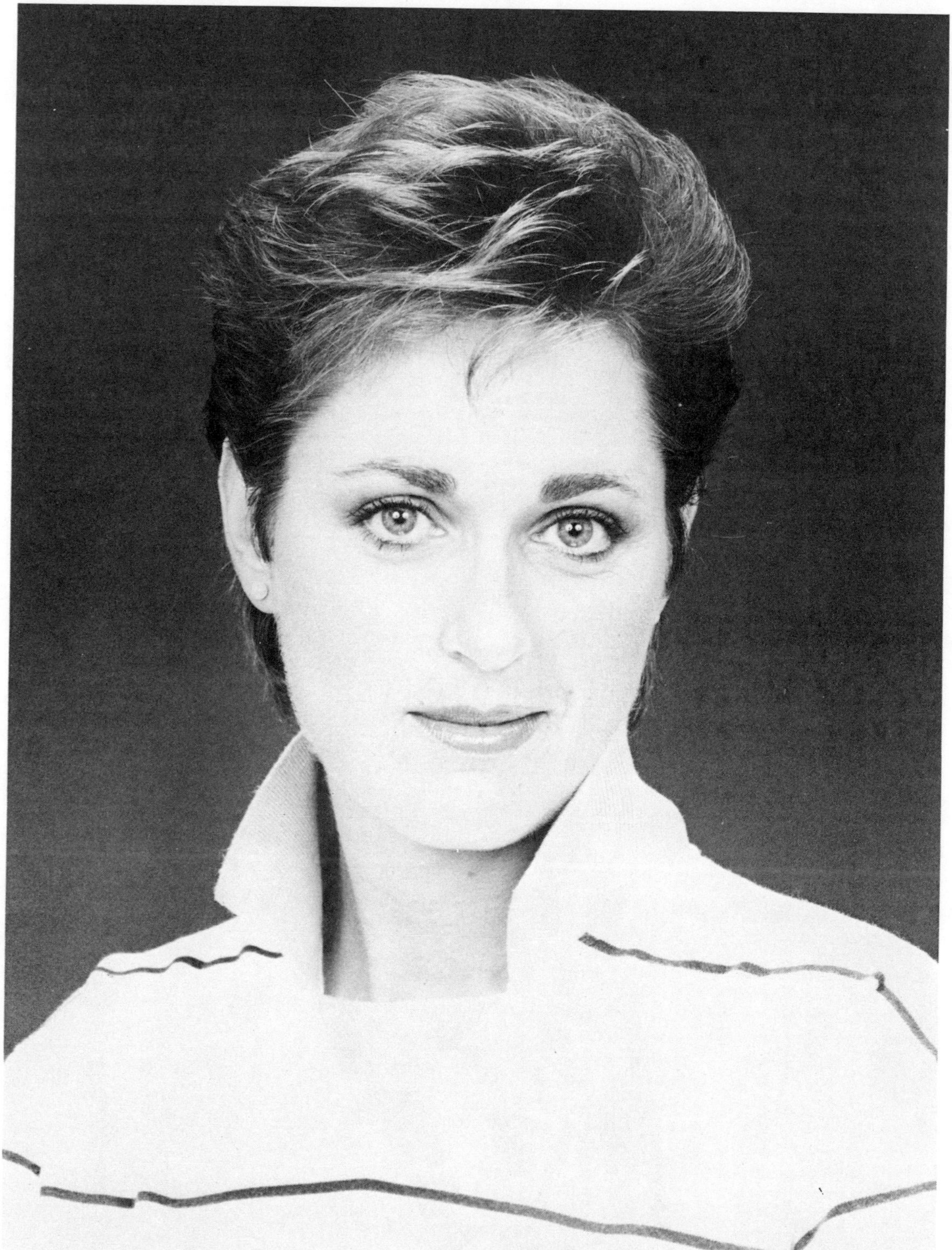

MUFFIN SPENCER-DEVLIN

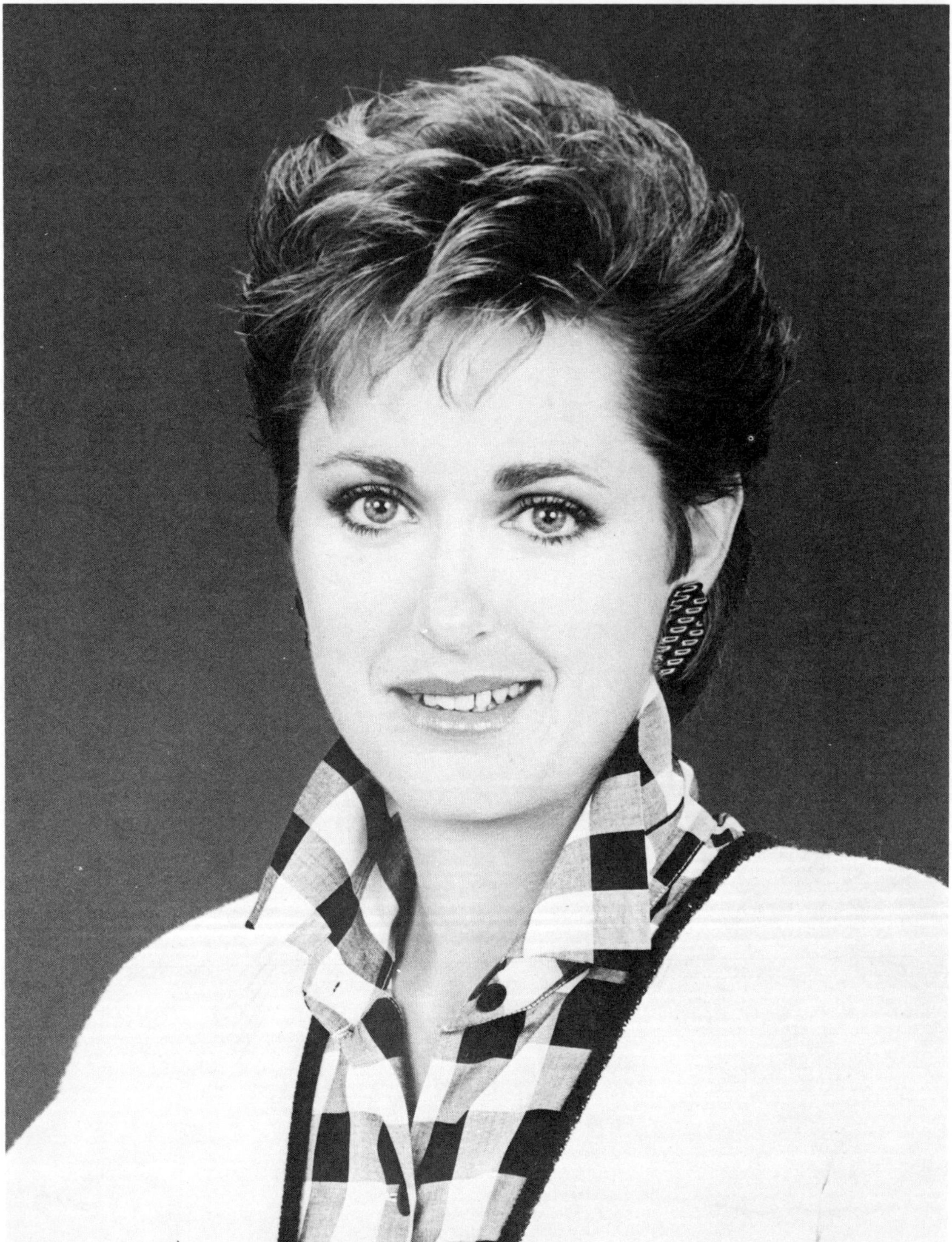

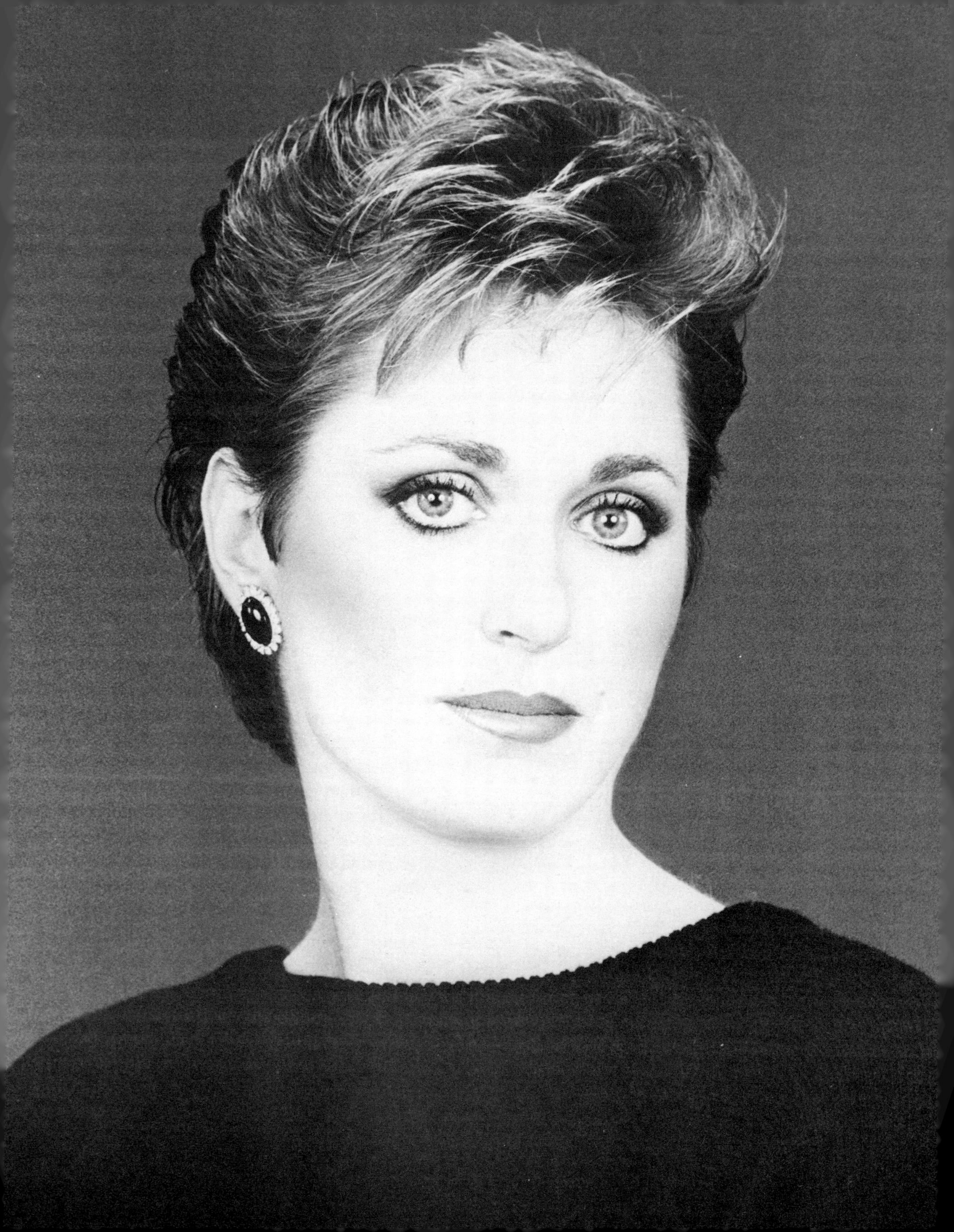

Muffin Spencer-Devlin, who, as a relative newcomer to professional golf (she joined the LPGA tour in 1979), has let no grass grow under her feet. Her success came gradually until 1984, when she tripled her 1983 earnings, almost equaling her total career take that year. Muffin's beauty tips are as applicable for the office worker as they are for the sportswoman.

On this particular day Muffin has to pace herself for an early-morning practice session on the golf course, followed by lunch with her manager, another business meeting the same afternoon, and finally an evening out. So a few quick-fix makeup maneuvers are an essential part of her schedule.

She starts her day with the barest hint of tinted moisturizer (over a sunblocker that has been applied to a cleaned and freshened face) and just lightly grazes her cheeks with a powdered blusher for a healthy outdoors glow. To save time, Muffin chooses not to fuss with separate eyeshadow. Instead, she uses a brown pencil to line her bottom lids right at the lash base and then blends some brown from the same pencil across her upper lids. A few feathery strokes with her mascara wand to bring her lashes into prominence make the final touch she needs to get just enough eye definition for the morning light. Then a few dabs of subtly tinted gloss at her lips—and *voilà!* Muffin has the perfect sportsworthy face. A similar look will take you just as beautifully through eighteen holes of golf or a brisk morning jog through the park.

But Muffin has only minutes to make her casual look a lot more businesslike for

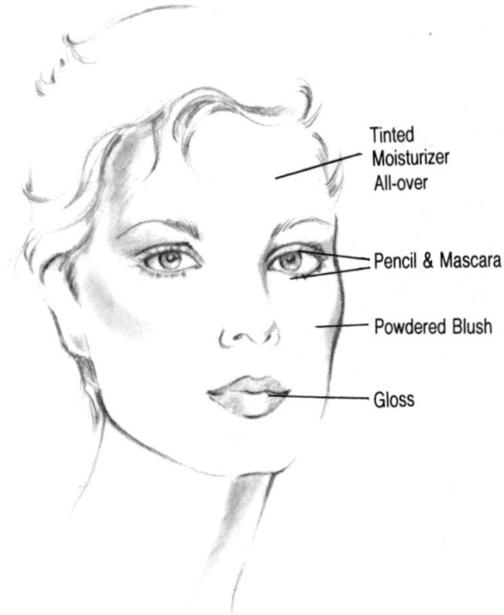

the next segment of her day. Enter the quick face fix-up.

- She freshens her face with a cotton pad dampened with skin toner, smooths on a second light coat of tinted moisturizer, deepening the color ever so slightly, and then blends a speck of concealer cream under her eyes until it melds into her skin tone.
- Now she dabs the outer edges of her upper eyelids with a touch of plum eye shadow, enhancing the brown that is already there. She blends it with her applicator sponge until you almost can't see it—a step that takes seconds but gives her eyes depth.
- With her brown pencil, she draws a not so smooth line right along the lash

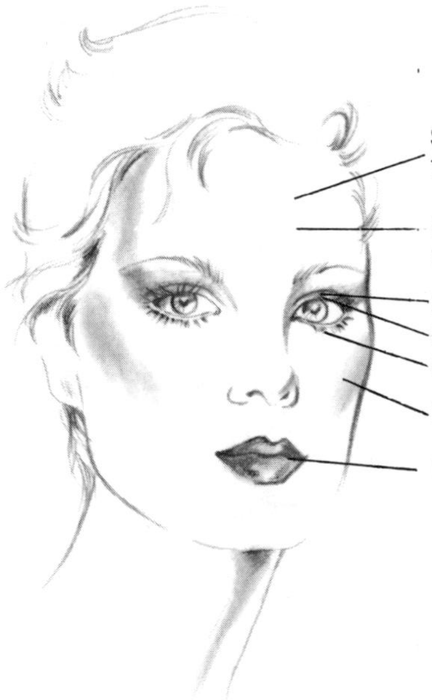

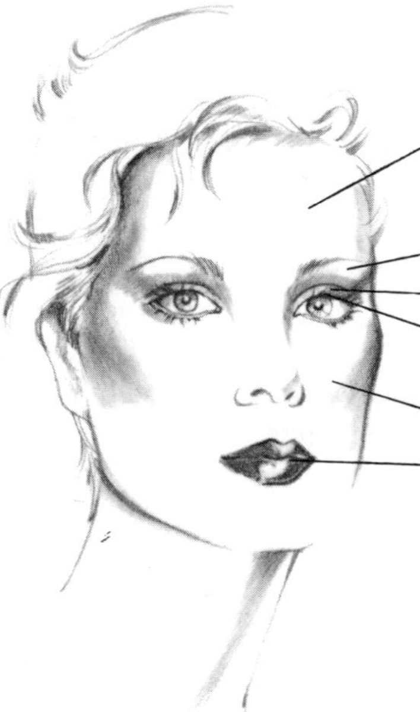

base of her upper lids. Then, with the applicator sponge from her eye shadow pack, she smudges the unevenness of the pencil line into a hazy rim, which, with the addition of a second coat of mascara, defines the shape of her eyes and makes her lashes appear a lot thicker than they actually are.

- Finally, after barely grazing her forehead, nose, and chin with powder for a polished look without shine, she colors her lips with lipstick and freshens her blusher, heightening the cheek color a bit with two or three swipes of the blusher brush.

The evening's festivities call for makeup rather more dramatic than businesslike, especially since Muffin's preference for understated dressing leads her to essentially unadorned basic black. But here she is with barely enough time to get home and change, let alone start her face from scratch.

Fortunately she doesn't have to. The only "foundation" she has been using all along is her tinted moisturizer. Now she simply adds a few dots of liquid foundation, spread with a slightly damp sponge, to get the silky-smooth look she likes her complexion to have for evenings.

- After setting her liquid base with a touch of translucent powder, primarily at her forehead, nose, and chin, she applies more blusher. This time she intensifies the color and sweeps it upward toward her hairline to define her cheekbones.
- Working with the eye design she created earlier, she leaves the original brown shadow (applied with her pencil

that morning) in place and deepens the plum eye shadow added just before lunch. Now she has only to highlight her brow bones with the lightest shade in her eye shadow pack.

- Her eyeliner goes on just as quickly and easily because she doesn't have to draw a new line. Instead, she whips out her black soft pencil and, in a series of quick, short strokes, traces over the brown eyeliner, smudging the results for a wonderful smoky look.
- Finally, she adds two more coats of mascara to her lashes and applies her lipstick, dabbing it lightly with lip gloss for a seductive shine.

Within minutes Muffin has created a radiant face for her evening out that looks as though she had spent hours before her mirror. You, too, can get a similar result in record time if you follow a few basic guidelines.

- Cleanse and moisturize your face properly at bedtime, and you'll wake up with little to do before applying that minimal morning makeup when you're rushing to stay on schedule.
- Don't let your lack of dexterity (real or imagined) bog you down when doing your eyes. Line them as much to make your lashes look thicker as to define their shape. You shouldn't even try for a perfectly smooth line. To do so is truly a waste of time when you'll be smudging it anyway for the best effect. Do try to get the liner down to the lash base, even if you wind up with a broken line, which you can blend with your applicator. In other words, aim with the pencil for your lashes, not above them.
- The softer the pencils you use, the more readily the color or shading will glide on. If you feel inept with eyeliner, you may find the thicker pencils easier to handle for this purpose. Hold your lid *slightly* taut from the outer corner while you gently glide the pencil along the rim with the other hand, in one long stroke or several short ones, whichever is more comfortable.

I don't know of a better place to apply the "less is more" principle than with makeup for the office, active sports, or casual outdoors occasions. Make it your golden rule of grooming, and you'll always have a basis for the many faces you want to present to the world. And you can create them in a flash, even when you have to dash.

ELEVEN

YOUR INSIDE TRACK TO EXPERTS

Must you live in or near a fashion capital to find top-notch professional grooming guidance? Not according to a former client of mine who moved to a small community where her husband had taken over a medical practice. After dealing with such major concerns as how and where they'd live and their children's schooling, Cynthia fretted over three somewhat lesser issues about the move from New York that nevertheless mattered a lot to her: Where in that seemingly "provincial" atmosphere would she find good tennis, a good, all-around fitness program, and a good hairdresser—not necessarily in that order?

Today Cynthia laughs at those worries. "There's no one more provincial, I learned, than a big-city dweller who thinks the world begins and ends within the city limits," she said when she came to see me during a recent trip to New York.

The social life of her small community, she noted, centers largely on the country club. There she found more than enough good tennis and a well-equipped gym, enabling her to work out several times a week. And through one of her doubles partners she eventually located a hairdresser whose work she likes.

"It took us awhile to get our act together, but we're quite a team now," Cynthia added, stressing newfound conviction that with a little research and patience you can find competent professional grooming help almost anywhere.

She's so right! In this age of instant global communication with satellite telecasts and women everywhere reading *Cosmo, Bazaar, Vogue,* and other fashion and beauty magazines published here and abroad, gone are the days when trends took months and years to filter down to the masses.

Admittedly, certain populations may take longer than others to adopt new ideas on a broad scale. But almost every community, large and small, has innovators who employ the latest techniques in their fields. You just have to ferret them out.

The very best method for choosing the right hairdresser, whether you live in the smallest hamlet where you have to travel to a neighboring town to find more than one salon or in a major urban center with hundreds to choose from: Ask an acquaintance whose hair you admire where she has it cut and styled *and by whom.* A salon's good reputation doesn't necessarily mean every hairstylist on its staff will give you the results you want.

If you don't admire anyone's hair at the moment, keep looking and keep your antenna up. Tune in to hairdos you see in restaurants and supermarkets, en route to work, or while jogging through the park—wherever you go. When you see a style you like, even if it's not your look but one that appears to have been well conceived and executed, don't be shy. March right up to the woman wearing it and ask for her hairdresser's name. She'll be so flattered you'll probably make her day.

Another possible avenue: Advertising and public relations agencies and commercial photographers often hire highly skilled hairstylists for photo assignments, fashion shows, and so on. Usually these individuals also work out of salons and accept private clients. Perhaps you know someone at one of these agencies who would be willing to recommend one or two people. Maybe even a phone call "cold" will get you a couple of names.

No matter where the recommendations come from, collect a few, if you can, just in case one or another doesn't pan out. Obviously, if a name pops up more than once from different sources, that's the stylist to try first.

Your initial visit should always focus on a consultation. I don't usually charge for consultations, but some hairstylists do, as is only fair if you expect a half hour or so of their time. Actually a consultation fee can work in your favor. When you pay for a stylist's time, you're entitled to it, and therefore, you tend not to feel guilty or rushed. On the other hand, if the hairdresser charges for consultations, it might just pay you to let him or her do your hair. In that case, don't expect a half hour consultation first or your hairdo may get short shrift so that the next client is not kept waiting.

As a rule, I find that five or ten minutes allow quite enough time to steer a prospective client in the right direction, and I rarely, if ever, recommend a drastic change (requiring major cutting, coloring, or perming, for example) on a first visit. On that occasion, stick to a blow-dry and styling. Most hairstylists will understand perfectly why you'd want to acquaint yourself with their approaches to styling before trusting them with total control over your head.

If a hairdresser has a problem dealing with that wisdom, it may be your first sign that he or she is too temperamental and won't be easy to communicate with at any point. Then I'd recommend moving on to the next name on your list since clearly one of your major objectives in the first session is to open a line of communication with the hairstylist—not to choke it off. Obviously you want to use the opportunity to see how he or she will handle your hair. But you also want to know if this is someone you can talk to, someone who'll listen to what you say. After all, you're the client. You're the one who's buying the service. And you're the one who can always go elsewhere if you're not pleased.

It's only fair for you to remember that this early your hairdresser is working with another hairdresser's cut, putting him or her at a distinct disadvantage. And since you want the best results he or she can produce, it behooves you to help your new stylist in every way short of saying, "Go ahead and do whatever you want," before you feel ready to do so.

One sure way to help both of you: Resist the inclination to walk into the salon when your hair looks positively desperate for attention. On the contrary, you'll be setting a higher standard if you take the trouble to shampoo and style your hair, making it look as good as it can. If you wander in there with your hair looking a mess, almost anything a hairdresser will do has to look great by comparison—hardly a test of his or her skills.

Also, introduce yourself to the hairstylist before you change into a smock or have your hair shampooed. Consultations work best with dry hair. When I meet a client for the first time, I want as many clues as possible to her expectations before we even begin, and I like to see her in street clothes.

If she's wearing a pin-striped suit, she wants something very different from the woman in a leather mini, belted at the hip. I can also tell a lot from a client's shoes, believe it or not. The lady wearing Charles Jourdan pumps wants to be fussed over and needs a hairstyle with a lot more chic than the woman in spiked heels and fishnet hose who obviously likes trendy things. And the woman in espadrilles or penny loafers clearly favors the swingy line of a bob to complement her pretty look. Even jewelry can be a giveaway. You send quite a different message flashing a five-karat diamond ring from the one you convey with plastic neon bracelets.

In short, dress according to the image you project—or want to project—most of the time. If you live in suits and dresses, don't walk into a salon for the first time wearing running or tennis shoes even though they're more comfortable for walking to work. Or if you do spend countless hours wearing sweatsuits and other sports gear, this is no time to dress up like a mannequin in Bergdorf's window.

But even before you enter the salon, you can do a lot to help a hairstylist help you. If there was ever a time when a picture was truly worth a thousand words, this is one. Pore through as many magazines as it takes to find a couple of photos depicting hairstyles on the order of what you'd like.

Since you're not shooting for a major change at this point, be reasonably sure the styles you clip can be created from the hair you have. By now you should know pretty well what you can or can't expect of your hair in its present state. And by all means, let the hairdresser know you don't expect a carbon copy of the photographed styles. Instead, you'd like to move away from the style you're wearing more toward the look suggested in the clippings and are willing to accept modifications dictated by your hair type.

You'll know at once from his or her sigh of relief that your eminently reasonable request has an appreciative audience. In return, you'll get a more satisfactory result, which is why you're there in the first place.

Magazine clippings become even more important, however, when you're ready to make a major change, such as cutting, coloring, or perming. If you have any doubts whatever, your hairdresser will know instantly just how radical a change you'd need to achieve the look you want with your hair in its present condition.

Finding a skin care and makeup professional is another matter entirely. Since women don't seek this kind of expertise as readily as they have their hair done, you won't find too many opportunities for the kinds of referrals you get in the hair department.

Still, if you do see someone whose makeup appears to have a professional touch, by all means ask her where she learned to apply it. She'll be just as flattered as the woman who sent you to her hairdresser and may lead you to an expert in the field.

Other potential avenues to advice on skin care and makeup are also worth exploring, especially if you'd like a whole new face design as part of your easy-to-maintain and distinctive look. After all, why should you rely on guesswork in this area any more than you'd cut your own hair?

Start by checking out department store cosmetics counters that usually offer a free makeup lesson with a purchase. Admittedly the instructor may have been demonstrating food processors in the same store the week before. And more than likely she or he was trained hurriedly for this stint as a makeup "expert" whose primary goal is to sell as much product as possible. But here's where a little homework on your part comes in handy. Hang around one or two of those counters to see what is done for other people. And if the salesperson is a woman, notice how her makeup is applied. Chances are if she acquired a flair for doing her own, she could pass that on to you.

Pharmacies and health and beauty aid outlets also have personnel trained to advise you or show you how to use makeup for the most dramatic effects.

And watch your local newspaper for ads announcing impending visits by representatives from the various cosmetic lines. These are bona fide makeup artists and skin care specialists who tour the country in behalf of various companies to stage clinics and workshops, usually right at the department stores.

Other possibilities:

- Does your hair salon employ a facialist who can give you creative makeup advice? Or perhaps the salon's manager can steer you toward a good skin care and makeup center in your area. These have mushroomed all over the country in recent years. Some are simply well-established retail cosmetics chains; others are to skin care what health clubs are to body fitness.
- If an ad agency or other local business led you to a hairdresser, the very same source may also lead you to a makeup artist who is willing to come to your home if she or he doesn't have a studio. Make an evening of it. Invite a few friends to share the benefits and defray the cost. Keep the group small—to no more than three or four—so you'll each get a fair share of personal attention.

At the very least you'll have a wonderful evening's entertainment. But I'd be disappointed if you didn't seize this opportunity to wind up with a new, freshfaced look you love, one you can play up or down in mere minutes for a whole gamut of interesting effects.

Of course, to be truly fabulous, that versatile new face of yours needs a stunning and equally versatile hairstyle to frame it, one you can maintain with relatively little fuss and only occasional professional attention. The hairstylist whose skills and attitude inspire your confidence is just the person to help you attain that goal. But he or she can't succeed without your significant contribution. So to help your hairstylist help you gain maximum control over your hair

- Get to know your hair and understand its potential and limitations.
- Give your hair a sporting chance to keep you looking terrific by keeping it healthy in every way possible.
- Take advantage of all the right styling tools and other aids to assume the kind of control over your hair you want. But . . .
- Don't try to wander too far from your hair's natural inclination so you don't find yourself with major maintenance headaches.
- Don't look for instant proficiency in handling your hair or the tools you need to maintain it if you never did that much with it before. And . . .
- Above all, don't get discouraged when a particular method or look doesn't pan out as you thought it would. If one approach doesn't work, another one will. It's that simple. Creating a whole

new style can and should be an exciting challenge. But you must be patient. For just as it often takes up front cash to earn big bucks, you must be willing to invest the time it takes for trial and error and to practice techniques. Only then will you save time and still get the kind of high performance results you want.

TWELVE

QUESTIONS AND ANSWERS

Do you have a particularly frustrating hair problem? If so, you're not alone. Almost everybody has at least one at any given time. And while I can't address every dilemma individually here, I can do the next best thing by discussing the questions that pop up most often—in a hundred different ways. More than likely you'll find your problem among them—perhaps not precisely as you might have stated it but with a solution you can apply anyway.

1. **Q.** Why is my hair so dull and drab-looking, and what can I do about it?

   A. Your lackluster hair could come from any one or a combination of factors. Chances are, it's too dry from overexposure to sun, wind, and other elements, from incorrect use of appliances, or from neglect after it's been permed or colored.

   If it's oily and dull, your hair might be coated with a film of grime mixed with residues from the overly zealous use of styling aids, inadequate shampooing, or incomplete rinsing.

   The obvious solution is to figure out which of these

you're doing wrong and stop doing it—or do the opposite. That's not to say you should curtail your outdoor activities. But if your problem comes from dry hair, you must counter the effects of the elements, especially if your hair is colored or permed, if you ever hope to put some luster back into it. Give your ailing tresses some intensive care—and a little extra TLC—with hot-oil treatments or with intense conditioning treatments. If you're already doing one or the other occasionally, step up the pace for a while.

Of course, your problem may be simply a dull, drab color. If so, consider one of the myriad approaches to color enhancing (see Chapter 9). In some instances you can rev up your hair color without really changing it and get not only shine but extra body as well.

Finally, if you can't account for the drabness of your hair in any other way, check with your physician to see if you have an internal disorder, perhaps from a hormonal imbalance or nutritional deficiency.

2. **Q.** Can hair spray and other styling aids ruin my hair?
A. Since they wash out with every shampoo, assuming you wash your hair several times a week, it's highly unlikely.

3. **Q.** My mother shampoos her hair once a week and insists I'm ruining mine by washing it more often. Is she right?
A. Not according to today's standards, with women as active as they are. Shampoo as often as necessary to keep your hair clean and free of excess oil. The oilier your scalp and the more you perspire, the more you'll probably feel the need to shampoo—perhaps every day or even twice a day at times. But your mother's attitude doesn't surprise me. She grew up at a time when weekly shampoos were common since women, for the most part, weren't as multidimensional as they are today. During the fifties and sixties many struggled to keep hairdos intact between weekly trips to the salon. For them, shampooing more than once a week was as unthinkable as shampooing only once a week is to you.

4. **Q.** Is it really necessary to lather up twice every time you shampoo?
A. When that weekly shampoo had to handle not only dirt and oils but gallons of lacquer and other stiffening agents women used to keep their hairstyles in place, two latherings with each shampoo made lots of sense. Not so today if you shampoo daily or several times a week. It actually depends on how dirty or oily your hair and scalp feel. Sometimes you may want to, but as a rule, I'd say lathering twice is a waste of time and might even prove to be overly drying.

5. **Q.** My hair is so dry and I have a

million split ends. How can I cure this condition?

A. There is no "cure" for dry hair, split ends, or any other hair damage. Damaged hair simply must grow out. But until it does, you can make it look, feel, and behave a lot more like healthy and manageable hair.

For starters, get rid of those split ends by having a good trim. Then begin at once to develop a sound haircare program. Pay particular attention to regular use of the right instant conditioners and intense conditioning treatments for your hair type (See Chapters 3 and 4). They'll help detangle your wet hair which will go a long way toward curtailing new breakage. In addition, they'll help smooth the cuticle layer.

Above all, don't abandon your hair care routine once you think you have the problem under control. If you want healthy, manageable hair permanently, a hair maintenance regimen must become a permanent part of your grooming ritual.

6. **Q.** Conditioning always leaves my hair limp and makes it oily within a few hours. Is there a way to avoid this problem and still condition my hair?

A. The symptoms you describe are typical of, but by no means exclusive to, fine hair. Be sure you're using the right conditioners—instant as well as intense. For fine, limp hair that oils up fast, you want conditioners with extra body. They contain less of the moisturizing agents that tend to encourage oiliness.

Then, in applying conditioners, avoid your scalp, and be sure to rinse thoroughly. Even after conditioning, which tends to make hair feel slippery, if cleaned and rinsed adequately, your hair will squeak just a little when run between your forefinger and thumb.

If none of that works for you, first apply your conditioner, comb it through with a wide-tooth comb, then shampoo only once. Although the shampoo will remove the conditioner on the surface of your hair, your hair shafts will have benefited sufficiently from its effects.

7. **Q.** What can I do to improve my fine, thin hair?

A. For one thing, although you may believe conditioners will make your hair droop even more than it does on its own, resist the inclination to avoid them. Diligent attention to hair care, including regular conditioning, is your first and foremost step toward bringing that fine, thin hair of yours to peak performance level. Look for shampoos and conditioners formulated for extra body. (See Question No. 6.) The best ones for you are those that have extra protein. Studies have shown that protein, which is added in bulk form to hair care products, often helps make hair look and feel thicker.

A permanent wave for body also could be extremely helpful if your hair is suitable for perming (see Chapter 8).

And any one of a variety of tinting techniques can provide yet another body-building option (see Chapter 9).

Finally, mousses can be your hair's best friend since they'll increase its stylability but are so light they won't overpower it.

8. **Q.** Will regular use of heat-inducing appliances such as blow-dryers and curling irons damage my hair?
A. Not if you use them correctly. But be sure to choose appliances from reputable manufacturers, bearing the Underwriters Laboratories approval seal.

9. **Q.** I've always been under the impression that the more you brush your hair, the better. But lately I've been hearing the opposite. Which is it—good for your hair or bad?
A. I like brushing for several reasons: It helps keep your hair clean by removing dirt and other foreign particles between shampoos. It spreads the oils more evenly through your hair, fostering its shine. It helps stimulate the scalp. And it's gentler than combing for removing tangles from *dry* hair.

But in this instance, as in some others, you can get too much of a good thing. Brushing too hard or too often can irritate the scalp and contribute to hair breakage or split ends. So forget about doing a vigorous hundred strokes a night, and just brush your hair daily as needed. (See Chapter 5 for the type of hairbrush I recommend for dry hair.)

10. **Q.** Will backbrushing or backcombing damage my hair?
A. Not if they're done properly on hair that's in good condition in the first place. In both procedures hair should be handled gently—not packed in tightly like the teased heads of the sixties (see Chapter 5 for instructions).

11. **Q.** Will my hair grow faster if I cut it often?
A. The notion that frequent cutting will make your hair grow is an old wives' tale. But getting a good trim at regular intervals will help your hair look and feel thicker and healthier because you'll almost never have damaged ends.

12. **Q.** What can I do about a haircut that doesn't work for me?
A. Here's where a good rapport with your hairdresser counts most. Don't procrastinate because you're afraid of offending him or her. Go back at once, but try to convey your disappointment without laying blame. What difference does it make at this point whether your hairdresser goofed or you failed to communicate your desires adequately? What matters now is getting a look you can handle and live with until it grows into a look you like. And remember, *it will grow*—as much as a half inch a month! So what you

want now is this individual's full and amiable cooperation.

Even short hair can be altered somewhat since reshaping doesn't necessarily require drastic cutting. On the other hand, you may need only a little advice and perhaps a few styling instructions on how to make this look work for you.

13. **Q.** Is there any way I can judge how my hair will take to a perm without going through the whole process and risk hating the results?
A. Yes! Just as you'd do a strand test before applying haircolor, have a test curl done on one small section at an inconspicuous area of your head.

14. **Q.** Assuming I plan to do both, which comes first: a haircut or a perm?
A. I first perm the hair in most cases. To see why, let's look at basketball star Nancy Lieberman's hair for a moment. She needed a cut but also wanted more body in her hair, which meant doing the permanent wave on larger rods. Had I first cut her hair, I would have had to use smaller permanent wave rods, which would have produced tighter curls, not a body wave.

15. **Q.** If you perm first and cut afterward, won't much of the perm wind up on the salon floor?
A. Not really, because you're perming the entire length of the hair—from root to end—and changing the all-over curl pattern. Once your hair is permed, the cut is totally different from what it would have been before the perm because you have a totally different head of hair to work with.

16. **Q.** What should I do if my permanent wave turns out too tightly curled?
A. Professionals have methods for relaxing the curl, but this should be attempted only if your hair is in good condition.

17. **Q.** Can I both color and perm safely?
A. Yes, but it's better for your hair if you wait a couple of days between the two processes. And *always* first perm, then color! Permanent wave solutions are stronger than most coloring agents. So if you color first, the perm could fade your new shade.

18. **Q.** If my hair is already color-treated, can I get a perm without ruining the color?
A. Sure. But use a permanent wave solution that's specially formulated for color-treated hair.

Also, if you have fine hair with highlights, and you want to perm for more volume and body, you'll do well to confine your fresh highlight touch-ups to the hairline areas around your face and to your crown. Let your back and nape section grow in to your natural shade (if it has highlights), and then perm there.

19. **Q.** What can I do to tone down highlights that have become so light

they contrast sharply with my natural hair color?

A. Apply a semipermanent hair-coloring agent (see Chapter 9) several shades lighter than your natural color over your entire head of hair. Since semipermanent coloring agents can't lighten hair, your natural shade will remain the same. You'll still have highlights, but they'll be subtle.

20. **Q.** I swim a great deal and hate to wear a bathing cap. What are the risks to my hair, and how can I protect it?

A. Most swimmers have to deal with excessively dry hair and scalp, and those with permed or color-treated hair who swim in chlorinated pools have an added risk: A variety of chemical interactions could throw a greenish cast into their hair color.

For the dry hair problem, the remedies recommended for lackluster hair in Question No. 1 will help considerably. Also, try to rinse your hair with fresh water after swimming in salt or chlorinated water. Many facilities have beach- and poolside showers, making it easy to do so.

21. **Q.** I realize some hair loss is normal, but can you tell me how much "normal" is?

A. Normal hair loss can range from twenty to sixty hairs a day. But you could lose less at certain times and more during high-stress periods. If you experience what seems abnormal hair fall over an extended time, I'd recommend consulting a dermatologist.

The final question wrestles with problem solving of a totally different kind. Ironically, it challenges the basic premise that inspired my hair care and grooming philosophy in the first place: that cosmetic improvements have the potential to enhance your lot in life dramatically, so you shouldn't take them lightly, nor should you have to struggle to attain them.

Assuming that you've absorbed much of the information contained in these pages and will implement that which pertains to you in order to derive the pertinent benefits, *can you really expect a meaningful impact on your well-being and on the way you live?*

I can only answer that the relationship between your appearance and your future is fraught with possibilities. What you make of it is up to you. I'm not suggesting that new approaches to grooming will solve all your problems. I can't even promise they'll solve all your beauty problems. But if I ever had any doubts that dramatic cosmetic improvements can influence a person's life, they vanished a few years ago when a major national magazine aimed at women asked the hair-coloring users among its readers to tell in an essay contest whether tinting their hair (among the most visible alterations one can effect) actually changed their lives. And if so, how so?

The very idea piqued my interest for obvious reasons, so I followed up on the results, which startled even me. That the overall response came back a resounding yes seemed almost insignificant compared with some of the other developments.

Women from all over the country had ferreted out the magazine's relatively small contest announcement. Though it offered rather modest rewards, even for the top prize, they took the time and trouble to share their experiences, often revealing highly personal details. Clearly those experiences made such a dramatic impact that the respondents were delighted at the opportunity to tell their stories despite the low-win or no-win risk.

Most stated that coloring their hair, often accompanied by cutting and restyling, started a whole chain of actions and reactions that promoted changes for the better in their lives. Those changes emanated from their own vastly improved self-images, the way others perceived them, or both.

In telling "How Haircoloring Changed or Improved My Life," respondents credited this cosmetic alteration with rekindling the spark in humdrum or troubled marriages, instigating major career advancements, and encouraging them to return to school, lose huge amounts of weight, assert themselves, or take other self-enhancing steps to improve their emotional health. One woman actually said her color change started a series of events that pulled her out of a severe chronic depression that had often landed her in the hospital.

But the letter that really knocked me out presented living proof that just knowing how terrific you look does wonders for your self-esteem and can upgrade other facets of your life. It came from a woman who, though she had lost her eyesight many years earlier, was lecturing before women's clubs and other organizations throughout the southern United States.

At her husband's suggestion she colored her "mousy gray" hair. "Wow! What a difference it made in my self-confidence," she wrote. Although she hadn't seen her own reflection for years, she said, "I realize *others* look at me all the time." And referring to her expanded program of speaking engagements, she added, "I know my hair looks great every time I stand before a group [and] feeling good about oneself inside and out is an important part of my philosophy."

I hope it also has become an important part of *your* philosophy—if it wasn't before. And with this book I sincerely hope that I've helped you to take a big step toward living that philosophy, beginning with a beautiful head of high performance hair.

INDEX